Evidence-based Hypertension

Edited by

Cynthia D Mulrow
Professor of Medicine
The University of Texas Health Science Center at San Antonio
Audie L Murphy Memorial Veterans Hospital
San Antonio, Texas, USA

BMJ
Books

© BMJ Books 2001
BMJ Books is an imprint of the BMJ Publishing Group

All rights reserved. No part of this publication may be reproduced,
stored in a retrieval system, or transmitted, in any form or by any
means, electronic, mechanical, photocopying, recording and/or
otherwise, without the prior written permission of the publishers.

First published in 2001
by BMJ Books, BMA House, Tavistock Square,
London WC1H 9JR
www.bmjbooks.com

British Library Cataloguing in Publication Data

A catalogue record for this book is available from the British Library

ISBN 0-7279-1438-3

Cover by BCD Design Ltd, London
Typeset by FiSH Books
Printed and bound in Spain by GraphyCems, Navarra.

Contents

Contributors

Jennifer Moore Arterburn
Veterans Evidence-based Research,
Dissemination, and Implementation
Center (VERDICT)
Audie L Murphy Memorial Veterans
Hospital
San Antonio, Texas, USA

David Cherney
Resident in Internal Medicine
Department of Medicine
Mount Sinai Hospital-University
Health Network
University of Toronto
Toronto, Ontario, Canada

Robert L Ferrer
Assistant Professor of Family Practice
Department of Family Practice
The University of Texas Health
Science Center at San Antonio
San Antonio, Texas, USA

Finlay A McAlister
Assistant Professor and AHFMR
Population Health Investigator
Division of General Internal Medicine
University of Alberta Hospital
Edmonton, Alberta, Canada

Cynthia D Mulrow
Professor of Medicine
Divisions of General Medicine
and Geriatrics
The University of Texas Health
Science Center at San Antonio
Division of General Internal Medicine
Audie L Murphy Memorial Veterans
Hospital
San Antonio, Texas, USA

Jane E O'Rorke
Assistant Professor of Medicine
Division of General Medicine
The University of Texas Health
Science Center at San Antonio
San Antonio, Texas, USA

Raj Padwal
Clinical Research Fellow
Division of General Internal Medicine
University of Alberta Hospital
Edmonton, Alberta, Canada

Michael Pignone
Assistant Professor of Medicine
Department of Internal Medicine
University of North Carolina
Chapel Hill, North Carolina, USA

W Scott Richardson
Associate Professor of Medicine
The University of Texas Health
Science Center at San Antonio
Veterans Evidence-based Research,
Dissemination and Implementation
Center (VERDICT)
Audie L Murphy Memorial Veterans
Hospital
San Antonio, Texas, USA

Stacey Sheridan
Primary Care Research Fellow
Department of Internal Medicine
University of North Carolina
Chapel Hill, North Carolina, USA

Sharon E Straus
Assistant Professor of Medicine
Department of Medicine
Mount Sinai Hospital-University
Health Network
University of Toronto
Toronto, Ontario, Canada

Karen Stamm
Veterans Evidence-based Research,
Dissemination, and Implementation
Center (VERDICT)
Audie L Murphy Memorial Veterans
Hospital
San Antonio, Texas, USA

Glossary: How we defined the terms

We use the following definitions for the evidence-based medicine terms in this book. The definitions are taken from *Clinical Evidence* compendium, published in December 1999 by the BMJ Publishing Group and the American College of Physicians-American Society of Internal Medicine.[1]

Absolute risk. This is the probability that an individual will experience the specified outcome during a specified period. It lies in the range 0 to 1. In contrast to common usage, the word "risk" may refer to adverse events (such as myocardial infarction), or desirable events (such as cure).

Absolute risk reduction. The absolute difference in risk between the experimental and control groups in a trial. It is used when the risk in the control group exceeds the risk in the experimental groups, and is calculated by subtracting the absolute risk in the experimental group from that of the control group. This figure does not give any idea of the proportional reduction between the two groups; for this, relative risk reduction is needed.

Attributable risk. Measure of how much of the disease burden could be eliminated if the exposure were eliminated. Alternatively, the rate of a disease or other outcome in exposed individuals that can be attributed to the exposure.

Case control study. A study design that examines a group of people who have experienced an event (usually an adverse event) and a group of people who have not experienced the same event, and looks at how exposure to suspect (usually noxious) agents differed between the two groups. This type of study design is most useful for trying to ascertain the cause of rare events, such as rare cancers.

Cohort study. A non-experimental study design that follows a group of people (a cohort), and then looks at how events differ among people within the group. A study that examines two cohorts, one that has been exposed to a suspect agent or treatment, and one that has not been exposed, is useful for trying to ascertain whether exposure is likely to cause specified events (often adverse). Prospective cohort studies that track participants forward in time are more reliable than retrospective cohort studies that look back in time to ascertain whether or not participants were exposed to the agent in question.

Confidence interval. The 95% confidence interval (CI) would include 95% of results from studies of the same size and design. This is close but not identical to saying that the true size of the effect has a 95% chance of falling within the confidence interval. If the 95% CI for a relative risk or an odds ratio crosses 1, the effect size is likely to lie in a range where risk is either increased or decreased.

Control. In a randomized controlled trial, the control refers to the participants in its comparison group. They are allocated either to placebo, to no treatment, or to the standard treatment.

Incidence. The number of new cases of a condition occurring in a population over a specified period of time.

Meta-analysis. A statistical technique that summarizes the results of several studies in a single weighted estimate, in which more weight is given to results from larger studies.

Morbidity. Rate of illness but not death.

Mortality. Rate of death.

Odds ratio. One measure of treatment effectiveness. It is the odds of an event happening in the experimental group, expressed as a proportion of the odds of an event happening in the control group. The closer the odds ratio is to one, the smaller the difference in effect between the experimental intervention and the control intervention. If the odds ratio is greater (or less) than one, then the effects of the treatment are more (or less) than those of the control treatment. Note that the effects being measured may be adverse (e.g., death or disability) or desirable (e.g., survival). When events are rare, the odds ratio is analogous to the relative risk, but as event rates increase, the odds ratio and relative risk diverge.

Placebo. A biologically inert treatment given to the control participants in trials.

Randomized controlled trial. A trial in which participants are randomly assigned to two or more groups: one (the experimental group) receiving the intervention that is being tested, and the others (the comparison or control groups) receiving an alternative treatment or placebo. This design allows assessment of the relative effects of interventions.

Relative risk. The number of times more likely (relative risk greater than 1) or less likely (relative risk less than 1) an event is in one group compared with another. It is analogous to the odds ratio when the events are rare and is the ratio of the absolute risk for each group.

Relative risk reduction. The proportional reduction in risk between experimental and control participants in a trial. It is the complement of the relative risk (1-relative risk).

Sensitivity. The chance of having a positive test result given that you have a disease.

Statistically significant. The findings of a study are unlikely to be due to chance. Significance at the commonly cited 5% level (P=0.05) means that the observed result would occur by chance in only 1 in 20 similar studies. Where the word "significant" or "significance" is used without qualification in the text, it is being used in this statistical sense.

Systematic review. A review in which all the trials on a topic have been systematically identified, appraised, and summarized according to predetermined criteria. It can, but need not, involve meta-analysis as a statistical method of adding together and numerically summarizing the results of the trials that meet minimum quality criteria.

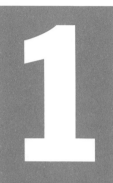

CHAPTER 1

A guide to this book

Karen Stamm
Jennifer Moore Arterburn

About the authors

How content is organized

How we located the evidence

How we rated the evidence

Final thoughts

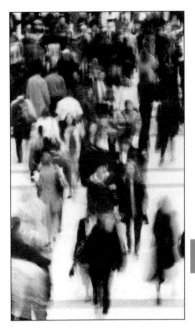

About 20 percent of the population will have hypertension at some point in their lives. This book is dedicated to people with this lifelong condition and the clinicians who care for them.

The rapidly changing landscape of hypertension research has unearthed many new treatment options for this silent, but serious, condition. May this book help clinicians evaluate these options accurately and efficiently, to the good of patient care.

About the authors

In the fall of 1998, BMJ Publishing Group approached us about writing a practice-oriented textbook for primary care clinicians on managing hypertension. We agreed that the book should summarize all available research evidence that clinicians need to care for hypertensive patients. We agreed to interpret the data to make them meaningful and useful and that we'd advise readers about the quality and quantity of the evidence supporting our findings. We intended that the book be practical, creative, and innovative—a helpful model for other evidence-based textbooks.

The authors are all academic clinicians who treat patients with hypertension in their general medicine practices. They share similar philosophies, which emerged as the chapters took shape. Obviously, they advocate a practice of basing clinical decisions on sound evidence. They believe that clinicians and patients should make clinical decisions as partners when possible and that treatment should be tailored to patients' unique circumstances. They advocate self-care for patients and continuous learning for themselves.

As technical writers, we were privileged to contribute throughout the entire editorial process. It was our first textbook. We tried to serve as advocates for readers and patients. Only you can judge if we succeeded in molding a monumental assortment of important information into a compact book that is easy to read and navigate.

We'd like to acknowledge other contributors:

- Molly Harris, our medical librarian extraordinaire, who devised no fewer than 11 literature search strategies that uncovered approximately 10 000 potentially relevant citations for the authors and verified more than 900 citations to ensure accurate references

- Dr Scott Richardson, our colleague, who from the project's inception offered creative ideas about the book's structure, content, and graphic presentation

- Linn Morgan and David Mullins, our valued administrative assistants, who lent a hand whenever we needed it with their trademark professionalism and good humor

- Mary Banks at BMJ Publishing Group, who guided us with a light hand and encouraging spirit

- Authors of the hundreds of studies and systematic reviews we reviewed, whose work provided the basis for our summarized findings

- Editors and authors of *Clinical Evidence: A Compendium of the Best Available Evidence for Effective Health Care, Issue 3,*[1] which served as an invaluable model and source of information.

 ## How content is organized

Although the chapters vary greatly in the type of evidence presented, each shares several universal elements:

- Clinical questions introduce various concise, discrete sections within chapters.

- Example clinical scenarios with patients introduce each chapter and are resolved.

- Summary bottom lines summarize actions suggested by the available evidence and its quality.

- Boxes, tables, and figures enhance key information.

- The type of evidence reviewed for each chapter, how it was located, and the authors' critique of its quality are noted.

- Accurate references are provided.

How we located the evidence

English citations dealing with humans were identified from 1990 to October 1999 from MEDLINE, The Cochrane Library, EMBASE, and PsycINFO online bibliographical databases; references of pertinent articles and reviews; *Clinical Evidence: A Compendium of the Best Available Evidence for Effective Heath Care, Issue 3,*[1] and experts. An update search was conducted on PubMed in June 2000.

We conducted 11 literature searches that identified more than 10 000 citations using subject headings unique to the individual online databases and specific textwords. The searches covered the following subject areas:

- Risk and prognosis
- Diagnosis and accuracy
- Patient decisions
- Treatment of hypertension
- Treatment of specific comorbid conditions, such as migraines and gout
- Adverse effects and contraindications of specific antihypertensive agents
- Management of hypertension
- Refractory hypertension, urgencies, and emergencies
- Patient adherence
- Hypertension in pregnancy
- Secondary hypertension

The search strategies used to identify systematic reviews and clinical trials were taken from the *Cochrane Reviewers' Handbook.*[2] Strategies used to identify therapy, diagnosis, etiology, and prognosis articles were taken from the book *PDQ: Evidence-based Principles and Practice.*[3] Detailed descriptions of the searches are available upon request.

How we rated the evidence

Grading the evidence is a tricky business. Not only are there numerous quality scales, but people take various approaches to applying them. We decided the imperfect, but reasonable, course was for each author to use the same scale, developed by the British National Health Service's Centre for Evidence-based Medicine (Table 1.1).[4] This scale, developed 20 years ago and revised in 1998, appears in other evidence-based textbooks.

Although the authors found the scale feasible, helpful, and challenging, they found themselves with the herculean task of applying it to a huge amount of hypertension literature. They found it was not applicable to all of the identified relevant evidence and that it was sometimes inadequate in capturing important nuances in qualities of evidence. They also found that the scale focused primarily on methodological quality of research evidence and that their evidence-based judgments relied heavily on assessing whether the clinical outcomes were important and large in size.

Table 1.1. Evidence grading scale[a] adapted from the Centre for Evidence-based Medicine.[4]

Level of evidence	Therapy, etiology, harm	Prognosis	Diagnosis
1a	Systematic review of multiple consistent trials.	Systematic review of multiple consistent inception cohort studies or a clinical practice guideline validated with a test set.	Systemative review with multiple consistent Level 1 diagnostic studies or a clinical practice guideline validated on a test set.
1b	Individual randomized trial with narrow confidence interval.	Inception cohort study with 80% or greater follow-up.	Independent blind comparison of patients from an appropriate spectrum of patients, all of whom have undergone both the diagnostic test and the reference standard.
1c	Strong consistent evidence of major benefit or harm before a therapy was introduced followed by strong absolutely consistent evidence of the opposite effect after a therapy was introduced.	Strong consistent evidence of major benefit or harm before a therapy was introduced followed by strong absolutely consistent evidence of the opposite effect after a therapy was introduced.	A diagnostic finding whose specificity is so high that a positive result rules in the diagnosis and a diagnostic finding whose sensitivity is so high that a negative result rules out the diagnosis.
2a	Systematic review of multiple consistent cohort studies.	Systematic review of either consistent retrospective cohort studies or consistent untreated control groups in trials.	Systematic review of multiple consistent diagnostic studies Level 2 or greater.

Table 1.1 continued. Evidence grading scale[a] adapted from the Centre for Evidence-based Medicine.[4]

Level of evidence	Therapy, etiology, harm	Prognosis	Diagnosis
2b	Individual cohort study or randomized trial with confidence intervals and/or less than 80% follow-up.	Retrospective cohort study or follow-up of untreated control patients in a trial or clinical practice guideline not validated in a test set.	Independent blind or objective comparison; or Study performed in a set of nonconsecutive patients or confined to a narrow spectrum of study individuals (or both), all of whom have undergone both the diagnostic test and the reference standard; or A diagnostic clinical practice guideline not validated in a test set.
2c	"Outcomes" research	"Outcomes" research	
3a	Systematic review of multiple consistent case-control studies.		
3b	Individual case-control study.		Independent blind or objective comparison of an appropriate spectrum, where the reference standard was not applied to all study patients.

[a]*The full scale includes grading levels 4 and 5 for rating evidence that has serious flaws or that represents expert opinion without critical appraisal of evidence.*

To show you how we graded the evidence, we devised and employed throughout the book a shorthand method that we use to code the levels of evidence for the studies we reviewed.

- For diagnosis, we use Dx:L__ ("L" stands for "level." Next to the "L" will be a number from 1 to 5, possibly followed by a letter denoting more specificity about the level. Use the table above as a guide.)
- For prognosis, we use Pr:L__
- For therapy, we use Tx:L__
- For etiology, we use E:L__
- For harm, we use H:L__

When we cite multiple references that are different levels, we indicate the multiple levels as follows: "Dx:L1, L2" or "Dx:L1, L3" or "Dx:L1, L2, L3."

 ## Final thoughts

We're all avid readers as well as writers. We tried to design a book that would appeal to us if we happened upon it on a bookshelf or a website. The questions we asked ourselves most frequently were, "Would you read this?" "Would you understand this?" and "Would you expect to find that information here?"

To meet the needs of hurried and harried clinicians, we tried to organize information so that you can learn what you need at the moment. If you're in a hurry to get to the bottom line of particular questions, you can read just the list at the end of each chapter for a summary of major clinical findings. When you take time to explore a large question (chapter) in more depth, peruse the chapter contents page to learn the smaller questions the author addresses. It's easy to read about a discrete issue or to read the whole chapter. Do you want to know the quality of the evidence behind a recommendation or finding? Find those details in boldface within the text. Do you want to know about the magnitude of observed effects? Look for relative risks and odds ratios and their confidence intervals peppered throughout the text.

Lastly, we wanted the book to be a convenient reference, small in size, and light in weight, albeit not lightweight in content!

 ## References

1. *Clinical evidence: a compendium of the best available evidence for effective health care. Issue 3* (June). London, England: BMJ Publishing Group, 2000.

2. *The Cochrane reviewers' handbook*, ver. 4.0. Appendix 5c: Optimal search strategy for RCTs. In: The Cochrane Library, Issue 3, 2000. Oxford: Update Software.

3. McKibbon A, Eady A, Marks S. *PDQ: evidence-based principles and practice.* Hamilton, Ont.; St. Louis: B.C. Decker, 1999.

4. Levels of evidence and grades of recommendations. In: *Centre for evidence-based medicine.* 1999. [cited 2000 Aug 15]. Available from: URL: http://cebm.jr2.ox.ac.uk/docs/levels.html.

CHAPTER 2

What is this person's blood pressure?

Finlay A McAlister
Sharon E Straus

Is accurate blood pressure measurement important?

How should we measure blood pressure in the clinic?

What interferes with accurate blood pressure measurement?

What is the white-coat effect?

How well does clinic measurement reflect "true" blood pressure?

How many readings and visits are needed to diagnose hypertension?

Should we recommend home self-measurement?

Should we recommend ambulatory blood pressure monitoring?

Summary bottom lines

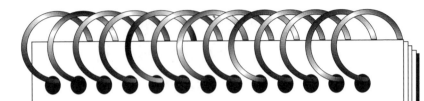

Patient Notes

Mr Hi Anxiety, age 55, accountant

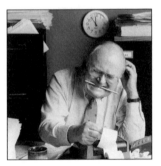

- Nonsmoker
- No family history of premature atherosclerotic disease
- Feels well
- Takes no medications on a regular basis

Reason for visit

- Routine yearly check-up

Clinical findings

- BP 160/110 mm Hg in the right arm sitting
- Examination otherwise normal

Clinical question

How do we most accurately and feasibly measure "true" blood pressure in adults?

Is accurate blood pressure measurement important?

There are many reasons we should routinely and accurately measure blood pressure in all adults. First, elevated blood pressure is a common finding that does not have specific clinical manifestations until target organ damage develops. Second, elevated blood pressure confers substantial risk of cardiovascular disease, particularly when it coexists with other risk factors such as diabetes, dyslipidemia, and tobacco use. Third, the incidence of cardiovascular events in people with elevated blood pressure can be reduced with appropriate drug therapy. Fourth, detecting and treating elevated blood pressure before onset of target organ damage is cost effective.[1] Fifth, systematically underestimating blood pressure denies large numbers of people access to potentially life-saving and morbidity-preventing therapy. For example, consistently underestimating diastolic blood pressure by 5 mm Hg could reduce the number of individuals appropriately identified as eligible for antihypertensive therapy by almost two-thirds.[2] Sixth, systematically overestimating blood pressure substantially increases numbers of individuals who receive inappropriate diagnostic labels and treatment recommendations. For example, consistently overestimating diastolic blood pressure by 5 mm Hg could more than double the number of individuals diagnosed with hypertension and significantly increase health care costs.[2] Seventh, whether the seemingly simple act of diagnosing and initiating therapy for "hypertension" causes significant psychosocial harm in and of itself is controversial. Observational studies from the 1970s and 1980s suggest that such diagnostic labeling is associated with worsened self-perceived health, increased psychosocial stress, and increased absenteeism from work,[3-7] but more recent observational studies suggest no or minimal psychosocial sequelae.[8,9](H: L2)

How should we measure blood pressure in the clinic?

We need to pay careful attention to technique when measuring blood pressure in order to maximize the accuracy and reliability of this diagnostic test. Numerous bodies have published guidelines for measuring blood pressure that are remarkably consistent (an infrequent finding with guidelines!). Recommendations adapted from the American Heart Association are outlined in Box 2.1.[10]

Box 2.1. Guides for accurate measurement of blood pressure.

- Seat the patient in a quiet environment with his or her bared arm resting on a support that places the midpoint of the upper arm at the level of the heart.

- Use a large cuff or estimate the circumference of the upper arm at the midpoint between the shoulder and elbow and select an appropriately sized cuff. The bladder inside the cuff should encircle 80% of the arm.

- Place the midline of the bladder over the arterial pulsation and wrap and secure the cuff snugly. The lower edge of the cuff should be 2 cm (1 in) above the antecubital fossa.

- Inflate the cuff rapidly to 70 mm Hg, and increase it by 10 mm Hg increments while palpating the radial pulse. Note the level of pressure at which the pulse disappears and subsequently reappears during deflation.

- Place the stethoscope earpieces into the ear canals, angled forward to fit snugly. Using the low-frequency position (bell), place the head of the stethoscope over the brachial artery pulsation.

- Inflate the bladder rapidly and steadily to 20 to 30 mm Hg above the level previously determined by palpation, then partially unscrew the valve and deflate the bladder about 2 mm/sec.

- Note the level of the pressure on the manometer at the first appearance of repetitive Korotkoff sounds (Phase I), at the muffling of sounds (Phase IV), and when they disappear (Phase V). Rate of bladder deflation should be no more than 2 mm per pulse beat.

- After the last Korotkoff sound is heard, deflate the bladder slowly for at least another 10 mm Hg to ensure that no further sounds are audible.

- Record the systolic (Phase I) and diastolic (Phase V) pressures rounded upwards to the nearest 2 mm Hg.

- Repeat measurement after the cuff's bladder has been completely deflated for at least 30 seconds.

Number of readings

The American Heart Association suggests averaging two readings in the same arm taken at least 30 seconds apart.[10] When these two values differ by more than 5 mm Hg, we follow the recommendations of the American Society of Hypertension and take additional readings until a stable level is reached.[11]

Measuring in one arm versus two

We try to measure blood pressure in both arms at initial assessment and subsequently use the arm with the higher pressure.[10] Simultaneously obtained bilateral direct arterial tracings have shown differences of 10 mm Hg or greater between arms in as many as 6% of people with hypertension.[12] (Dx: L2) It is generally accepted that blood pressure tends to be higher in the right compared to the left arm.[13]

Measuring seated versus supine

We found little difference between blood pressure measured in the supine and sitting positions as long as the arm is supported at heart level.

Virtually all national guidelines endorse measurement in the sitting position, and most of the large clinical treatment trials used this position.

Using large versus small cuff

Virtually all national guidelines now recommend using a large cuff for all patients. The use of a cuff too large for an individual's arm has little or no effect on measured blood pressure,[14,15] and the most frequent cause of incorrect blood pressure measurements is using an inappropriately small cuff.[16, 17]

Using mercury vesus aneroid sphygmomanometer

Although mercury sphygmomanometers are uncommonly used, they are the recommended gold standard for the indirect measurement of blood pressure. Popular aneroid sphygmomanometers require regular calibration and checks to avoid nonzeroed gauges, cracked face plates, and defective rubber tubing.[18] Checks show that a third or more of aneroid sphygmomanometers may be 4 mm Hg or more out of calibration, and up to 10% may be 10 mm Hg or more out of calibration.[19]

Korotkoff Phase IV versus Phase V for diastolic pressure

Some clinicians are confused about whether the Phase IV Korotkoff sound (muffling) or the Phase V Korotkoff (disappearance of sound) is most appropriate for measuring diastolic blood pressure.[20] Virtually all national guidelines endorse using the Phase V Korotkoff because it more closely matches diastolic pressure measured by direct arterial monitoring, is more reproducible between observers, and was used in the clinical trials that established benefits of antihypertensive therapy. Using the Phase IV Korotkoff is appropriate in pregnant women and in individuals with aortic insufficiency.

Being properly compulsive versus selectively rigorous

Busy clinicians can be discouraged by the time needed to meticulously measure blood pressure as recommended in guidelines. One approach is to reserve the "proper" compulsive method for patients who have known or newly detected hypertension, other cardiovascular risk factors, or target organ damage.[13] Since the utility and cost of compulsive versus selective rigor in blood pressure measurement has not been rigorously evaluated, we sagely refrain from sharing our personal recommendations.

What interferes with accurate blood pressure measurement?

Mistakes

In a survey of 114 physicians, none followed all of the recommended procedures for measuring blood pressure.[19] Common mistakes that were reported by more than 60% of the physicians are presented in Box 2.2.

2.Box 2.2. Common physician mistakes in blood pressure measurement.

- Using an inappropriately small cuff
- Failing to allow rest periods before measurements
- Deflating the cuff too fast
- Failing to measure the blood pressure in both arms
- Failing to palpate maximal systolic blood pressure before auscultation

---

Routine patient activities

Daily blood pressure levels vary substantially in most people. Lowest levels are when individuals are quietly resting or sleeping. Some everyday activities that may affect blood pressure are summarized in Table 2.1. Given these distorting influences, all guidelines recommend a minimum five minute rest period before measuring blood pressure.

Table 2.1. Effects of routine activities on blood pressure (adapted).[2]

Activity	Effect on blood pressure (mm Hg)	
	Systolic blood pressure	Diastolic blood pressure
Attending a meeting	↑20	↑15
Commuting to work	↑16	↑13
Dressing	↑12	↑10
Walking	↑12	↑6
Talking on telephone	↑10	↑7
Eating	↑9	↑10
Doing desk work	↑6	↑5
Reading	↑2	↑2
Watching television	↑0.3	↑1

Other patient, technique, and measurer factors

Numerous other factors that can affect the accuracy of blood pressure measurement are shown in Table 2.2. Although our literature search identified multiple studies that investigated potential sources of bias in the measurement of blood pressure, we selectively cite the studies that provided the highest level of evidence relevant to each factor.

Table 2.2. Factors that can interfere with the accuracy of blood pressure measurement.

Factor	Effect (measured blood pressure versus actual, mean values)		Highest quality of evidence[a]
	Systolic blood pressure	Diastolic blood pressure	
Patient factors			
Emotional extremes such as pain or marked anxiety	Variable ↑	Variable ↑	Level 5[13]
Eating or recent meal	↓ 1 mm Hg to no change	↓ 4 mm Hg to no change	Level 4[21]
Talking	↑ 17 mm Hg	↑ 13 mm Hg	Level 1[22]
Acute cold exposure	↑ 11 mm Hg	↑ 8 mm Hg	Level 2[23]
Physical activity	↓ 5 to 11 mm Hg for one hour or more	↓ 4 to 8 mm Hg for one hour or more	Level 4[24-26]
Bowel or bladder distension	↑ 27 mm Hg	↑ 22 mm Hg	Level 4[27]
Contraction of bowel or bladder sphincters	↑ 18 mm Hg	↑ 14 mm Hg	Level 4[27]
Paretic arm	↑ 2 mm Hg	↑ 5 mm Hg	Level 4[28]
White-coat effect	See text	See text	
High stroke volume	No effect	Variable ↓ (diastolic blood pressure can be zero)	Level 5[13]
Atherosclerotic arterial walls "pseudohypertension"	Variable ↑ or ↓	Variable ↑ or ↓	Level 4[29,30]
Smoking	↑ 10 mm Hg for 30 minutes or more	↑ 8 mm Hg for 30 minutes or more	Level 4[31]
Caffeine ingestion	↑ 10 mm Hg for 2 hours or less	↑ 7 mm Hg for 2 hours or less	Level 4[31]
Alcohol ingestion	↑ 8 mm Hg for 3 hours or less	↑ 7 mm Hg for 3 hours or less	Level 1[32]
Auscultatory gap	↓ up to 40 mm Hg	↑ up to 40 mm Hg	Level 5[33]
Soft Korotkoff sounds	Variable ↓	Variable ↑	Level 5[13]
Technique factors			
Supine versus sitting	No effect to ↑ 3 mm Hg if supine	↓ 2 to 5 mm Hg if supine	Level 1[34,35]

Table 2.2 continued. Factors that can interfere with the accuracy of blood pressure measurement.

Factor	Effect (measured blood pressure versus actual, mean values)		Highest quality of evidence[a]
	Systolic blood pressure	Diastolic blood pressure	
Arm position	↓ (or ↑) 8 mm Hg for every 10 cm above (or below) heart level	↓ (or ↑) 8 mm Hg for every 10 cm above (or below) heart level	Level 1[36]
Failure to support arm	↑ 2 mm Hg	↑ 2 mm Hg	Level 1[36]
Back unsupported	No effect to ↑ 8 mm Hg	↑ 6 to 10 mm Hg	Level 4[37, 38]
Patient's legs crossed	Variable ↑	Variable ↑	Level 5[39]
Too much pressure on stethoscope	No effect	Variable ↓	Level 5[14]
Bell versus diaphragm	[b]Minimal or no difference	[b]Minimal or no difference	Level 4 [37, 40–42]
Cuff too small	↓ BP 8 mm Hg	↑ BP 8 mm Hg	Level 1[43]
Leaky bulb valve	Variable ↓	Variable ↑	Level 4[44]
Cuff too large	↓ up to 3 mm Hg (no effect in most patients)	↓ up to 5 mm Hg (no effect in most patients)	Level 4[15]
Cuff not centered	↑ up to 4 mm Hg	↑ up to 3 mm Hg	Level 5[45]
Cuff over clothing	↑ up to 50 mm Hg	↑ up to 50 mm Hg	Level 5[13, 37]
Cuff too loose	Variable ↑	Variable ↑	Level 5[46]
Cuff deflation too fast	Variable ↓	Variable ↑	Level 5[13, 47]
Repeated cuff inflation (venous congestion)	Wide variability (from ↑ of 30mm Hg to ↓ of 14mm Hg)	Wide variability (from ↑ of 20mm Hg to ↓ of 10 mm Hg)	Level 5[13, 48]
Faulty sphygmomanometer	Variable effect	Variable effect	Level 5[13, 18]
Environmental noise	Unpredictable ↓	Unpredictable ↑	Level 5[13]
Measurer factors			
Expectation bias including end-digit preference	Rounding to nearest 5 or 10 mm Hg	Rounding to nearest 5 or 10 mm Hg	Level 1[49]
Impaired hearing	Unpredictable ↓	Unpredictable ↑	Level 5[13]
Time pressure of examiner	Unpredictable ↓	Unpredictable ↓	Level 5[50]
Parallax error	Variable ↑ or ↓	Variable ↑ or ↓	Level 5[13]

[a]*Level of evidence for diagnostic studies.*
[b]*Minimal or no differences are differences that are ± 1 mm Hg.*

What is the white-coat effect?

The white-coat effect is the phenomenon whereby blood pressures that are measured by medical personnel are elevated above usual levels. In normotensive individuals, there is generally little or no difference between clinic and usual blood pressures. However, discrepancies between clinic and usual blood pressure are consistently seen in patients with hypertension.[51-53] This so-called white-coat hypertension is more common in older than younger adults and in women than men.[54]

As many as 20% of patients diagnosed with hypertension based on clinic blood pressures have entirely normal ambulatory blood pressures. These so-called white-coat hypertensives include a small proportion (4%) of patients with very high clinic blood pressures that are 180/110 mm Hg or higher.[51, 55, 56] Although it is difficult to say with certainty in the absence of Level 1 diagnostic studies, up to 40% of patients with hypertension may demonstrate white-coat effects in excess of 20/10 mm Hg.[13, 57]

Reducing the white-coat effect

One way to reduce the white-coat effect is to recheck blood pressure at the end of the clinic visit to confirm the value obtained at the beginning of the visit. The degree of white-coat effect is most pronounced when the patient first enters the examination area and declines rapidly over time.[58]

Another method of reducing the white-coat effect is to have a nurse or technician measure the blood pressure. The white-coat effect is of smaller magnitude when medical professionals other than physicians measure blood pressure.[59, 60]

Diagnosing white-coat hypertension

There are no clear-cut, validated diagnostic criteria for white-coat hypertension. Differences between clinic and ambulatory blood pressure are highly variable over time,[41](Dx: L1) and white-coat hypertension cannot be diagnosed by clinical examination alone.

Individuals with white-coat hypertension do not necessarily exhibit anxious symptoms, tachycardia, or other manifestations of increased sympathetic activity.[56, 61-63] Following are clues that may suggest the presence of a white-coat effect: persistently elevated clinic blood pressures in the absence of hypertensive target organ damage; elevated clinic blood pressure with symptoms suggesting postural hypotension; and marked discrepancy between blood pressure readings obtained in clinic and other settings.

Cardiovascular risk of white-coat hypertensive versus normotensive patients

While the magnitude of the white-coat effect does not predict cardiovascular risk,[64](Pr: L1) we found conflicting evidence regarding whether patients with white-coat hypertension are at higher cardiovascular risk than normotensive individuals. Two large cohort studies failed to find any excess cardiovascular risk in patients with isolated white-coat hypertension.[65, 66](Pr: L1) On the other hand, cross-sectional studies have documented a higher prevalence of left ventricular hypertrophy in people with white-coat hypertension,[67-69] and three small cohort studies have suggested that white-coat hypertension is associated with structural and vascular changes in the carotid arteries and left ventricle similar to those seen with sustained hypertension.[70-72] (Pr: L1, L2) Moreover, many individuals with white-coat hypertension subsequently develop persistent hypertension.[73]

Whether lowering blood pressure in patients with purely white-coat hypertension reduces cardiovascular endpoints is unknown.

How well does clinic measurement reflect "true" blood pressure?

As pointed out by Reeves, "in clinical blood pressure measurement, we look through a series of dark glasses."[13] Assuming that our office measurement techniques are correct and that none of the factors outlined in Table 2.2 are operative, we may still have further sources of error. Indirect blood pressure measurements with a sphygmomanometer may not reflect the concurrent intra-arterial blood pressure and clinic blood pressures may not reflect the usual blood pressure of an individual over 24 hours.

Indirect versus direct blood pressure measurement

Even when indirect blood pressure measurements are correctly obtained, there may be substantial discrepancies between the Korotkoff sounds and corresponding intra-arterial readings. While indirect blood pressures correlate well with intra-arterial readings (correlation coefficients 0.94 to 0.98),[59] Korotkoff sounds neither appear nor disappear simultaneously with systolic and diastolic intra-arterial pressure readings. For example, Phase I Korotkoff sounds do not appear until an average of 3 mm Hg below the direct systolic blood pressure and the Phase V Korotkoff sounds disappear an average of 9 mm Hg higher than the direct diastolic blood pressure.[74, 75](Dx: L1) Such direct-indirect discrepancies are not equal in all patients; elderly patients with sclerotic arterial walls may have substantially higher indirect blood pressures than intra-arterial blood pressures (See "Pseudohypertension" in Table 2.2). Regardless, the available evidence that documents many deleterious effects of high blood pressure and many benefits of antihypertensive treatment is derived from studies that used indirect not direct blood pressure measurements.

Clinic versus usual blood pressure

Blood pressure varies markedly over time. Standard deviations of as much as 4 mm Hg systolic and 3 mm Hg diastolic have been observed in continuous arterial blood pressure readings taken over several minutes.[76] This phenomenon occurs because blood pressure varies with each heartbeat, particularly in patients with cardiac arrhythmias, and with the respiratory cycle.[45] Differences are even more pronounced when blood pressures in the same patient are measured on different days where standard deviations as high as 12 mm Hg systolic and 8 mm Hg diastolic have been observed.[76, 77] Moreover, blood pressures in the same patient may vary by as much as ± 15/12 mm Hg on separate days 5% of the time.[13]

Blood pressure generally falls with repeated measurement. This is attributable to the following two factors: habituation and regression to the mean. Habituation occurs as patients become more familiar with the examiner and the procedures of blood pressure measurement. Regression to the mean is the tendency for any high (or low) measurement to fall (or rise) towards the population mean when repeated. Thus, using a single measurement to define an individual's blood pressure would overdiagnose hypertension in 20 to 30% of the population.[13, 78] By the same token, relying on only one measurement will miss one-third of those who are truly hypertensive.[79]

 # How many readings and visits are needed to diagnose hypertension?

We found that there is no universally accepted number of visits necessary to establish a diagnosis of hypertension, but all national guidelines recommend multiple visits. Randomized trials that established the benefits of antihypertensive therapy generally used two or three blood pressure readings at two or more clinic visits to establish the diagnosis. Mathematical models suggest that the lowest rate of false positives and negatives occur if two blood pressure readings are taken at each of four visits. Numbers of visits required are higher for patients with borderline blood pressures and lower (as few as two) for patients with markedly abnormal blood pressures, multiple other cardiovascular risk factors, or target organ damage.[79] Table 2.3 summarizes specific recommendations regarding initial blood pressure level and frequency of follow-up that were made by a United States consensus national guideline panel.[80]

Table 2.3. Joint National Committee on Prevention, Detection, Evaluation, and Treatment of High Blood Pressure recommendations for follow-up based on initial blood pressure (adapted).[80]

Systolic blood pressure (mm Hg)	Diastolic blood pressure (mm Hg)	Recommended follow-up
< 130	< 85	Recheck in two years
130 to 139	85 to 89	Recheck in one year
140 to 159	90 to 99	Confirm within two months
160 to 179	100 to 109	Confirm within one month
≥ 180	≥ 110	Confirm within one week

Number of measurements needed to "confirm" diagnosis not stated.

Should we recommend home self-measurement?

Having patients take their own blood pressure at home holds advantages and disadvantages.

Advantages

Multiple readings can be obtained over a prolonged period of time, allowing better definition of true blood pressure. Because no medical personnel are involved, distortions due to the white-coat effect are eliminated. The specificity of self-measured blood pressure for detecting white-coat hypertension as defined by 24-hour ambulatory blood pressure monitoring was 85% in a study of 189 people with high clinic blood pressures.[81](Dx: L2) This high specificity suggests self-monitoring is a reasonable screening measure and a reasonable method for follow-up of presumed white-coat hypertension or for treated hypertensive patients with known white-coat effect.

Disadvantages

There is a greater potential for errors in blood pressure measurement due to inadequate patient training and the poor accuracy of many home electronic monitors.[51,82](Dx: L2) One study found that only one of 30 patients using a manual home blood pressure monitor adhered to correct protocol and that less than 70% of the self-reported blood pressure measurements were identical to those recorded simultaneously on an automated machine.[83] Of interest, differences between self-measurements and automated machine measurements occurred more frequently in patients with elevated blood pressures. Another study involving 1207 participants found there were substantial differences in self-measured blood pressure within the same individuals at different times of day.[84](Dx: L4)

Another disadvantage is a lack of certainty and consensus about the reference values for home self-monitoring. In a recent meta-analysis of 17 studies involving 5422 normotensive or untreated hypertensive participants, the average blood pressure on home monitoring was 115/71 mm Hg in normotensive people.[85] Defining hypertension as two standard deviations above the mean, home readings of greater than 135/85 mm Hg could be considered hypertensive.

Home blood pressure monitoring and patient outcomes

Unfortunately, large-scale prospective data relating home blood pressure levels with cardiovascular outcomes are scant. Preliminary data from a study of 1789 patients suggest home readings more closely correlate with cardiovascular mortality than clinic pressures.[86](Pr: L1) Most epidemiological and all clinical trial data on cardiovascular morbidity and mortality in hypertensive patients are derived from studies that used clinic, rather than home, blood pressure measurements. Self-measured home blood pressure levels correlate only moderately with 24-hour ambulatory blood pressure monitoring levels; sensitivity is modest (57%) for detecting white-coat hypertension.[81](Dx: L2)

In a randomized trial of 430 hypertensive patients randomized to home blood pressure management or usual care, mean changes in blood pressure at one year were nonsignificantly lower in the intervention group (systolic blood pressure: –3.2 mm Hg, 95% CI –6.7 to 0.2 mm Hg; diastolic blood pressure: –1.6 mm Hg, 95% CI -3.6 to 0.4 mm Hg).[87](Tx: L1b) Home blood pressure monitoring patients made 1.2 fewer (95% CI 0.8 to 1.7) hypertension-related office visits, and costs of care were lower in this group.(Tx: L1b)

Should we recommend ambulatory blood pressure monitoring?

Ambulatory blood pressure monitoring (ABPM) permits the noninvasive measurement of blood pressure over a prolonged period of time (usually 24 hours). First developed as a research tool in the early 1960s, it has become increasingly popular in assessing hypertensive individuals.

Advantages

ABPM provides a more reproducible estimate of an individual's blood pressure than clinic pressures. ABPM is not subject to the regression to the mean phenomenon seen with repeated measurements in the clinic.[88] ABPM is relatively free of side effects other than rare cases of olecranon bursitis, petechia, superficial thrombophlebitis, and neuralgia.[89-92] Blood pressure values from ABPM are better correlated with the presence of target organ damage than clinic blood pressures.[93, 94](Pr: L1, L4) Virtually all of these studies investigated the association between ABPM readings and left ventricular mass, a surrogate marker that strongly predicts future cardiovascular events.[53] Although the literature on the ability of ABPM to predict cardiovascular risk is not as large and consistent as that for clinic blood pressures, available data suggest that ABPM provides additional prognostic information above that derived from clinic blood pressures.[65, 66, 95-97](Pr: L1)

The accuracy of ABPM in predicting cardiovascular risk depends on the reproducibility of the blood pressure measurements that are obtained. The predictive power of ABPM appears limited to those people with mean ABPM readings varying less than 4/3 mm Hg between days;[93](Dx: L1) however, almost one-third of people undergoing ABPM demonstrate between-day differences in mean blood pressure that are 7 mm Hg or higher.[98](Dx: L1)

Disadvantages

ABPM is an expensive technology; total costs are estimated at $6 billion if ABPM were used routinely for diagnosing and managing hypertension in the United States.[53] Interestingly, in a recent study of 233 patients, multiple nonphysician-measured clinic blood pressures had high correlation coefficients with ABPM and were just as highly associated with albuminuria and left ventricular hypertrophy as ABPM.[99]

ABPM "dippers" and "nondippers"

Most people with essential hypertension are "dippers"; their mean nocturnal blood pressure is over 10 mm Hg lower than their mean daytime blood pressure. However, ABPM identifies a subgroup of people with hypertension who are "nondippers." Compared to "dippers," "nondippers" may exhibit higher rates of hypertensive target organ damage[100-102](Pr: L4) and increased cardiovascular morbidity and mortality,[66, 97, 103](Pr: L1) even after adjustment for age, sex, presence of other cardiovascular risk factors, and baseline blood pressures. We advise caution when applying this evidence because separating patients into "dippers" and "nondippers" is arbitrary (daytime-nocturnal blood pressure differences are normally distributed) and the reproducibility of dipping status is limited.[104] For example, in a study of 253 untreated hypertensive patients undergoing 48-hour ABPM, only 71% remained in the same classification group ("dipper" or "nondipper") on consecutive days.[105](Dx: L1)

Normal ABPM range

As with clinic blood pressure measurements, there is debate over the normal range for ABPM. In their most recent guidelines, the Joint National Committee on Prevention, Detection, Evaluation, and Treatment of High Blood Pressure (JNC VI) and the American Society of Hypertension chose values that were validated by a Level 1 prognostic study to represent the point at which hypertensive target organ damage begins to develop (Table 2.4).[80, 106, 107]

Table 2.4. American Society of Hypertension Definitions for ABPM (adapted).[107]

	Probably normal	Borderline	Probably abnormal
Systolic average			
Awake	< 135 mm Hg	135 to 140 mm Hg	> 140 mm Hg
Asleep	< 120 mm Hg	120 to 125 mm Hg	> 125 mm Hg
24 hour	< 130 mm Hg	130 to 135 mm Hg	> 135 mm Hg
Diastolic average			
Awake	< 85 mm Hg	85 to 90 mm Hg	> 90 mm Hg
Asleep	< 75 mm Hg	75 to 80 mm Hg	> 80 mm Hg
24 hour	< 80 mm Hg	80 to 85 mm Hg	> 85 mm Hg
Load[a]			
Systolic	< 15%	15 to 30%	> 30%
Diastolic	< 15%	15 to 30%	> 30%

[a]Load defined as the percentage of ambulatory blood pressure measurements above threshold (140/90 mm Hg awake and 120/80mm Hg nocturnal).

When ABPM should be used

Although using ABPM in all individuals suspected of being hypertensive would reduce the frequency of misdiagnosis, the cost and drain on available resources would be tremendous.[108] Thus, expert consensus suggests that ABPM is most useful under the following circumstances:[107]

- Suspected white-coat hypertension
- Apparent drug resistance
- Episodic hypertension
- Suspected autonomic dysfunction
- Hypotensive symptoms on antihypertensive therapy.

Several ongoing randomized trials are investigating the role of ABPM versus clinic blood pressures in monitoring hypertensive therapy. We found a randomized trial of 419 hypertensive participants that showed that following patients with ABPM rather than clinic blood pressures led to less intensive drug treatment with preservation of blood pressure control, left ventricular mass, and general well-being.[109](Tx: LI) The cost-effectiveness of this approach is still being investigated. Until several ongoing studies are complete, the strategy proposed by an ad-hoc panel of the American Society of Hypertension provides reasonable guidance for the clinician (Figure 2.1).[107]

Figure 2.1. American Society of Hypertension strategy for the use of ABPM (adapted).[107]

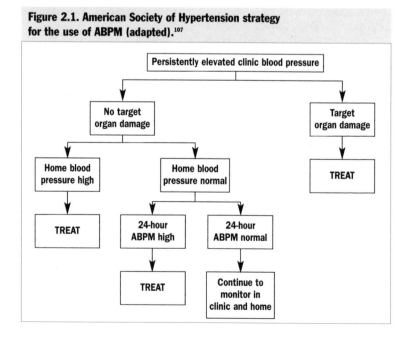

Both the Association for the Advancement of Medical Instrumentation and the British Hypertension Society have developed protocols for validating blood pressure measurement devices that should be reviewed if ABPM is being considered.[110, 111]

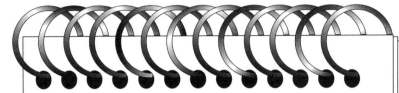

Patient Notes

Mr Hi Anxiety,

- Routine check-up
- BP 160/110mm Hg

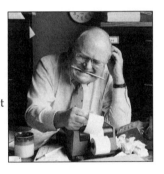

Recommendations

- Return to clinic twice in the next two months for repeat blood pressure checks
- Regular exercise and diet
- Obtain a home blood pressure monitor
- Bring monitor to next clinic visit for calibration
- Visit lab to get fasting lipid profile and glucose prior to next clinic visit

Clinician plan

- Take two blood pressure readings over the next two months following the complete protocol for accurate blood pressure measurement set forth in American Heart Association guidelines (Box 2.1).

Summary bottom lines

- To accurately measure clinic blood pressure, use the bell of the stethoscope and take two readings in the same arm at least 30 seconds apart. If the two values differ by more than 5 mm Hg, take additional readings until a stable level is reached; using a single measurement could over- or underdiagnose hypertension in 20 to 30% of the population. Use Phase V Korotkoff (disappearance of sound) when measuring diastolic blood pressure because it most closely matches true diastolic pressure. Use a large blood pressure cuff in all patients to avoid the possibility of using one too small, which is a common mistake. (Consensus opinions)

- Allow patients to rest before measuring blood pressure because common activities can cause substantial distortion. Evidence regarding specific factors that raise blood pressure levels and their magnitude of effect is generally weak. Some factors reported to increase systolic blood pressure levels by more than 10 mm Hg include talking, acute cold exposure, bowel or bladder distension or contracted sphincters, smoking during the previous 30 minutes, caffeine ingestion in the previous two hours, placing cuff over clothing, and repeated cuff inflation. (Generally Level 4 and 5 studies)

- Be meticulous in following guidelines for proper measurement particularly when patients have newly detected elevated blood pressure, cardiovascular target organ damage, or other risk factors or are receiving antihypertensive therapy. (Consensus opinion)

- The white-coat effect can raise blood pressure in excess of 20/10 mm Hg in up to 40% of patients. When this is suspected, recheck blood pressure at the end of a clinic visit, or have a nurse or technician measure blood pressure rather than the physician. (Consensus opinion)

- Take two blood pressure readings at each of four visits to yield the lowest rate of false positive and false negative diagnoses. (Mathematical models)

- Consider home self-measurement of blood pressure to help avoid overdiagnosis due to white-coat effects. Realize that whether patient measurement errors, inaccurate home monitors, and poor correlation between self-measured blood pressure and ABPM more than offset the potential benefits is unknown. (Consensus opinion)

- Consider ABPM for evaluating patients with suspected white-coat hypertension, apparent drug resistance, episodic hypertension, suspected autonomic dysfunction or hypotensive symptoms on antihypertensive therapy. (Consensus opinion)

We identified information for this chapter by searching MEDLINE from 1966 to 2000. We searched for English language and human-related literature relevant to the diagnosis of hypertension and white-coat hypertension. We used search hedges specifically designed to identify studies addressing diagnosis and accuracy. We screened approximately 1000 titles and/or abstracts to help identify the highest quality relevant information to include in this chapter.

References

1. Littenberg B. A practice guideline revisited: screening for hypertension. *Ann Intern Med* 1995; **122**:937-9.

2. Campbell NR, McKay DW. Accurate blood pressure measurement: why does it matter? *CMAJ* 1999; **161**:277-8.

3. Haynes RB, Sackett DL, Taylor DW, Gibson ES, Johnson AL. Increased absenteeism from work after detection and labeling of hypertensive patients. *N Engl J Med* 1978; **299**:741-4.

4. Mossey JM. Psychosocial consequences of labelling in hypertension. *Clin Invest Med* 1981; **4**:201-7.

5. Polk BF, Harlan LC, Cooper SP, *et al.* Disability days associated with detection and treatment in a hypertension control program. *Am J Epidemiol* 1984; **119**:44-53.

6. Bloom JR, Monterossa S. Hypertension labeling and sense of well-being. *Am J Public Health* 1981; **71**:1228-32.

7. Harlan LC, Polk BF, Cooper S, *et al.* Effects of labeling and treatment of hypertension on perceived health. *Am J Prev Med* 1986; **2**:256-61.

8. Moum T, Naess S, Sorensen T, Tambs K, Holmen J. Hypertension labelling, life events and psychological well-being. *Psychol Med* 1990; **20**:635-46.

9. Lefebvre RC, Hursey KG, Carleton RA. Labeling of participants in high blood pressure screening programs. Implications for blood cholesterol screenings. *Arch Intern Med* 1988; **148**:1993-7.

10. Perloff D, Grim C, Flack J, *et al.* Human blood pressure determination by sphygmomanometry. *Circulation* 1993; **88**:2460-70.

11. American Society of Hypertension. Recommendations for routine blood pressure measurement by indirect cuff sphygmomanometry. *Am J Hypertens* 1992; **5**:207-9.

12. Harrison JEG, Roth GM, Hines JEA. Bilateral indirect and direct arterial pressures. *Circulation* 1960; **22**:419-36.

13. Reeves RA. Does this patient have hypertension? How to measure blood pressure. *JAMA* 1995; **273**:1211-18.

14. Baker RH, Ende J. Confounders of auscultatory blood pressure measurement. *J Gen Intern Med* 1995; **10**:223-31.

15. Sprafka JM, Strickland D, Gomez-Marin O, Prineas RJ. The effect of cuff size on blood pressure measurement in adults. *Epidemiology* 1991; **2**:214-17.

16. Manning DM, Kuchirka C, Kaminski J. Miscuffing: inappropriate blood pressure cuff application. *Circulation* 1983; **68**:763-6.

17. Linfors EW, Feussner JR, Blessing CL, Starmer CF, Neelon FA, McKee PA. Spurious hypertension in the obese patient. Effect of sphygmomanometer cuff size on prevalence of hypertension. *Arch Intern Med* 1984; **144**:1482-5.

18. Bailey RH, Knaus VL, Bauer JH. Aneroid sphygmomanometers. An assessment of accuracy at a university hospital and clinics. *Arch Intern Med* 1991; **151**:1409-12.

19. McKay DW, Campbell NR, Parab LS, Chockalingam A, Fodor JG. Clinical assessment of blood pressure. *J Hum Hypertens* 1990; **4**:639–45.

20. McAlister FA, Laupacis A, Teo KK, Hamilton PG, Montague TJ. A survey of clinician attitudes and management practices in hypertension. *J Hum Hypertens* 1997; **11**:413–19.

21. Mader SL. Effects of meals and time of day on postural blood pressure responses in young and elderly subjects. *Arch Intern Med* 1989; **149**:2757–60.

22. Le Pailleur C, Helft G, Landais P, *et al*. The effects of talking, reading, and silence on the "white coat" phenomenon in hypertensive patients. *Am J Hypertens* 1998; **11**:203–7.

23. Scriven AJ, Brown MJ, Murphy MB, Dollery CT. Changes in blood pressure and plasma catecholamines caused by tyramine and cold exposure. *J Cardiovasc Pharmacol* 1984; **6**:954–60.

24. Kenney MJ, Seals DR. Postexercise hypotension. Key features, mechanisms, and clinical significance. *Hypertension* 1993; **22**:653–64.

25. Pescatello LS, Fargo AE, Leach CN Jr, Scherzer HH. Short-term effect of dynamic exercise on arterial blood pressure. *Circulation* 1991; **83**:1557–61.

26. Cleroux J, Kouame N, Nadeau A, Coulombe D, Lacourciere Y. Aftereffects of exercise on regional and systemic hemodynamics in hypertension. *Hypertension* 1992; **19**:183–91.

27. Szasz JJ, Whyte HM. Effect of distension of the bladder and of contraction of sphincters on blood pressure. *BMJ* 1967; **ii**:208–10.

28. Yagi S, Ichikawa S, Sakamaki T, Takayama Y, Murata K. Blood pressure in the paretic arms of patients with stroke. *N Engl J Med* 1986; **315**:836.

29. Messerli FH, Ventura HO, Amodeo C. Osler's maneuver and pseudohypertension. *N Engl J Med* 1985; **312**:1548–51.

30. Oliner CM, Elliott WJ, Gretler DD, Murphy MB. Low predictive value of positive Osler manoeuvre for diagnosing pseudohypertension. *J Hum Hypertens* 1993; **7**:65–70.

31. Freestone S, Ramsay LE. Effect of coffee and cigarette smoking on the blood pressure of untreated and diuretic-treated hypertensive patients. *Am J Med* 1982; **73**:348–53.

32. Potter JF, Watson RD, Skan W, Beevers DG. The pressor and metabolic effects of alcohol in normotensive subjects. *Hypertension* 1986; **8**:625–31.

33. Askey JM. The auscultatory gap in sphygmomanometry. *Ann Intern Med* 1974; **80**:94–7.

34. Netea RT, Smits P, Lenders JW, Thien T. Does it matter whether blood pressure measurements are taken with subjects sitting or supine? *J Hypertens* 1998; **16**:263–8.

35. Jamieson MJ, Webster J, Philips S, *et al*. The measurement of blood pressure: sitting or supine, once or twice? *J Hypertens* 1990; **8**:635–40.

36. Waal-Manning HJ, Paulin JM. Effects of arm position and support on blood–pressure readings. *J Clin Hypertens* 1987; **3**:624–30.

37. Cushman WC, Cooper KM, Horne RA, Meydrech EF. Effect of back support and stethoscope head on seated blood pressure determinations. *Am J Hypertens* 1990; **3**:240–1.

38. Viol GW, Goebel M, Lorenz GJ, Ing TS. Seating as a variable in clinical blood pressure measurement. *Am Heart J* 1979; **98**:813–14.

39. Rudy SF. Take a reading on your blood pressure techniques. *Nursing* 1986; **16**:46–9.

40. Prineas RJ, Jacobs D. Quality of Korotkoff sounds: bell vs diaphragm, cubital fossa vs brachial artery. *Prev Med* 1983; **12**:715–19.

41. Parati G, Omboni S, Staessen J, *et al*. Limitations of the difference between clinic and daytime blood pressure as a surrogate measure of the "white-coat" effect. Syst-Eur investigators. *J Hypertens* 1998; **16**:23–9.

42. Mauro AM. Effects of bell versus diaphragm on indirect blood pressure measurement. *Heart Lung* 1988; **17**:489–94.

43. Russell AE, Wing LM, Smith SA, *et al*. Optimal size of cuff bladder for indirect measurement of arterial pressure in adults. *J Hypertens* 1989; **7**:607–13.

44. Conceicao S, Ward MK, Kerr DN. Defects in sphygmomanometers: an important source of error in blood pressure recording. *BMJ* 1976; **i**:886–8.

45. Webb CH. The measurement of blood pressure and its interpretation. *Prim Care* 1980; **7**:637–51.

46. O'Brien ET, O'Malley K. ABC of blood pressure measurement. Technique. *BMJ* 1979; **ii**:982–4.

47. Campbell NR, McKay DW, Chockalingam A, Fodor JG. Errors in assessment of blood pressure: blood pressure measuring technique. *C J Public Health* 1994; **85**:S18–21.

48. O'Brien ET, O'Malley K. ABC of blood pressure measurement. The patient. *BMJ* 1979; **ii**:920–1.

49. Neufeld PD, Johnson DL. Observer error in blood pressure measurement. *CMAJ* 1986; **135**:633–7.

50. O'Brien ET, O'Malley K. ABC of blood pressure measurement. The observer. *BMJ* 1979; **ii**:775–6.

51. Pickering TG. Blood pressure measurement and detection of hypertension. *Lancet* 1994; **344**:31–5.

52. Pickering TG, James GD. Some implications of the differences between home, clinic and ambulatory blood pressure in normotensive and hypertensive patients. *J Hypertens* 1989; **7**(Suppl):S65–72.

53. Appel LJ, Stason WB. Ambulatory blood pressure monitoring and blood pressure self-measurement in the diagnosis and management of hypertension. *Ann Intern Med* 1993; **118**:867–82.

54. Myers MG, Reeves RA. White coat effect in treated hypertensive patients: sex differences. *J Hum Hypertens* 1995; **9**:729–33.

55. Inden Y, Tsuda M, Hayashi H, *et al.* Relationship between Joint National Committee–VI classification of hypertension and ambulatory blood pressure in patients with hypertension diagnosed by casual blood pressure. *Clin Cardiol* 1998; **21**:801–6.

56. Martinez MA, Garcia–Puig J, Martin JC, *et al.* Frequency and determinants of white coat hypertension in mild to moderate hypertension: a primary care–based study. Monitorizacion Ambulatoria de la Presion Arterial (MAPA)–Area 5 Working Group. *Am J Hypertens* 1999; **12**:251–9.

57. Staessen JA, O'Brien ET, Atkins N, Amery AK. Short report: ambulatory blood pressure in normotensive compared with hypertensive subjects. The Ad-Hoc Working Group. *J Hypertens* 1993; **11**:1289–97.

58. Mancia G, Bertinieri G, Grassi G, *et al.* Effects of blood–pressure measurement by the doctor on patient's blood pressure and heart rate. *Lancet* 1983; **ii**:695–8.

59. Ellis PJ, Marshall E, Ellis SJ. Which blood pressure? *Lancet* 1988; **ii**:902–3.

60. Mancia G, Parati G, Pomidossi G, Grassi G, Casadei R, Zanchetti A. Alerting reaction and rise in blood pressure during measurement by physician and nurse. *Hypertension* 1987; **9**:209–15.

61. Julius S, Jamerson K, Gudbrandsson T, Schork N. White coat hypertension: a follow-up. *Clin Exp Hypertens A* 1992; **14**:45–53.

62. MacDonald MB, Laing GP, Wilson MP, Wilson TW. Prevalence and predictors of white–coat response in patients with treated hypertension. *CMAJ* 1999; **161**:265–9.

63. Mansoor GA, McCabe EJ, White WB. Determinants of the white–coat effect in hypertensive subjects. *J Hum Hypertens* 1996; **10**:87–92.

64. Verdecchia P, Schillaci G, Borgioni C, Ciucci A, Porcellati C. Prognostic significance of the white coat effect. *Hypertension* 1997; **29**:1218–24.

65. Perloff D, Sokolow M, Cowan R. The prognostic value of ambulatory blood pressures. *JAMA* 1983; **249**:2792–8.

66. Verdecchia P, Porcellati C, Schillaci G, *et al.* Ambulatory blood pressure. An independent predictor of prognosis in essential hypertension [published erratum

appears in *Hypertension* 1995;**25**:462]. *Hypertension* 1994; **24**:793–801.

67. Cerasola G, Cottone S, Nardi E, *et al.* White-coat hypertension and cardiovascular risk. *J Cardiovasc Risk* 1995; **2**:545–9.

68. Verdecchia P, Schillaci G, Boldrini F, Zampi I, Porcellati C. Variability between current definitions of "normal" ambulatory blood pressure. Implications in the assessment of white coat hypertension. *Hypertension* 1992; **20**:555–62.

69. Weber MA, Neutel JM, Smith DH, Graettinger WF. Diagnosis of mild hypertension by ambulatory blood pressure monitoring. *Circulation* 1994; **90**:2291–8.

70. Zakopoulos N, Papamichael C, Papaconstantinou H, *et al.* Isolated clinic hypertension is not an innocent phenomenon: effect on the carotid artery structure. *Am J Hypertens* 1999; **12**:245–50.

71. Glen SK, Elliott HL, Curzio JL, Lees KR, Reid JL. White-coat hypertension as a cause of cardiovascular dysfunction. *Lancet* 1996; **348**:654–7.

72. Ferrara LA, Guida L, Pasanisi F, *et al.* Isolated office hypertension and end–organ damage. *J Hypertens* 1997; **15**:979–85.

73. Bidlingmeyer I, Burnier M, Bidlingmeyer M, Waeber B, Brunner HR. Isolated office hypertension: a prehypertensive state? *J Hypertens* 1996; **14**:327–32.

74. O'Brien E, Mee F, Atkins N, O'Malley K. Inaccuracy of the Hawksley random zero sphygmomanometer. *Lancet* 1990; **336**:1465–8.

75. Stolt M, Sjonell G, Astrom H, Hansson L. Factors affecting the validity of the standard blood pressure cuff. *Clin Physiol* 1993; **13**:611–20.

76. Reeves RA. A review of the stability of ambulatory blood pressure: implications for diagnosis of hypertension. *Clin Invest Med* 1991; **14**:251–5.

77. Reeves RA, Leenen FH, Joyner CD. Reproducibility of nurse–measured, exercise and ambulatory blood pressure and echocardiographic left ventricular mass in borderline hypertension. *J Hypertens* 1992; **10**:1249–56.

78. Birkett NJ. The effect of alternative criteria for hypertension on estimates of prevalence and control [published erratum appears in *J Hypertens* 1997;**15**:804]. *J Hypertens* 1997; **15**:237–44.

79. Perry HM Jr, Miller JP. Difficulties in diagnosing hypertension: implications and alternatives. *J Hypertens* 1992; **10**:887–96.

80. Joint National Committee on Prevention, Detection, Evaluation, and Treatment of High Blood Pressure. The sixth report of the Joint National Committee on Prevention, Detection, Evaluation, and Treatment of High Blood Pressure [published erratum appears in *Arch Intern Med* 1998;**158**:573]. *Arch Intern Med* 1997; **157**:2413–46.

81. Stergiou GS, Zourbaki AS, Skeva II, Mountokalakis TD. White coat effect detected using self–monitoring of blood pressure at home: comparison with ambulatory blood pressure. *Am J Hypertens* 1998; **11**:820–7.

82. Pickering TG, Cvetkovski B, James GD. An evaluation of electronic recorders for self–monitoring of blood pressure. *J Hypertens* 1986; **4**:S328–30.

83. Johnson KA, Partsch DJ, Rippole LL, McVey DM. Reliability of self–reported blood pressure measurements. *Arch Intern Med* 1999; **159**:2689–93.

84. Imai Y, Nishiyama A, Sekino M, *et al.* Characteristics of blood pressure measured at home in the morning and in the evening: the Ohasama study. *J Hypertens* 1999; **17**:889–98.

85. Thijs L, Staessen JA, Celis H, *et al.* Reference values for self–recorded blood pressure: a meta–analysis of summary data. *Arch Intern Med* 1998; **158**:481–8.

86. Ohkubo T, Imai Y, Tsuji I, *et al.* Home blood pressure measurement has a stronger predictive power for mortality than does screening blood pressure measurement: a population–based observation in Ohasama, Japan. *J Hypertens* 1998; **16**:971–5.

87. Soghikian K, Casper SM, Fireman BH, *et al.* Home blood pressure monitoring. Effect on use of medical services and medical care costs. *Med Care* 1992; **30**:855–65.

88. Myers MG, Haynes RB, Rabkin SW. Canadian hypertension society guidelines for ambulatory blood pressure monitoring [published erratum appears in *Am J Hypertens* 2000;**13**:219]. *Am J Hypertens* 1999; **12**:1149–57.

89. Mansoor GA, White WB. Olecranon bursitis associated with 24–hour ambulatory blood pressure monitoring. *Am J Hypertens* 1994; **7**:855–6.

90. White WB. The Rumpel–Leede sign associated with a noninvasive ambulatory blood pressure monitor. *JAMA* 1985; **253**:1724.

91. Bottini PB, Rhoades RB, Carr AA, Prisant LM. Mechanical trauma and acute neuralgia associated with automated ambulatory blood pressure monitoring. *Am J Hypertens* 1991; **4**:288.

92. Creevy PC, Burris JF, Mroczek WJ. Phlebitis associated with noninvasive 24–hour ambulatory blood pressure monitor. *JAMA* 1985; **254**:2411.

93. Palatini P, Mormino P, Santonastaso M, Mos L, Pessina AC. Ambulatory blood pressure predicts end–organ damage only in subjects with reproducible recordings. HARVEST Study Investigators. Hypertension and Ambulatory Recording Venetia Study. *J Hypertens* 1999; **17**:465–73.

94. Khattar RS, Senior R, Swales JD, Lahiri A. Value of ambulatory intra–arterial blood pressure monitoring in the long–term prediction of left ventricular hypertrophy and carotid atherosclerosis in essential hypertension. *J Hum Hypertens* 1999; **13**:111–16.

95. Khattar RS, Swales JD, Banfield A, Dore C, Senior R, Lahiri A. Prediction of coronary and cerebrovascular morbidity and mortality by direct continuous ambulatory blood pressure monitoring in essential hypertension [published erratum appears in *Circulation* 1999;**100**:1760]. *Circulation* 1999; **100**:1071–6.

96. Ohkubo T, Imai Y, Tsuji I, *et al.* Prediction of mortality by ambulatory blood pressure monitoring versus screening blood pressure measurements: a pilot study in Ohasama. *J Hypertens* 1997; **15**:357–64.

97. Staessen JA, Thijs L, Fagard R, *et al.* Predicting cardiovascular risk using conventional vs ambulatory blood pressure in older patients with systolic hypertension. Systolic Hypertension in Europe Trial Investigators. *JAMA* 1999; **282**:539–46.

98. Palatini P, Mormino P, Canali C, *et al.* Factors affecting ambulatory blood pressure reproducibility. Results of the HARVEST Trial. Hypertension and Ambulatory Recording Venetia Study. *Hypertension* 1994; **23**:211–16.

99. Jula A, Puukka P, Karanko H. Multiple clinic and home blood pressure measurements versus ambulatory blood pressure monitoring. *Hypertension* 1999; **34**:261–6.

100. Giaconi S, Levanti C, Fommei E, *et al.* Microalbuminuria and casual and ambulatory blood pressure monitoring in normotensives and in patients with borderline and mild essential hypertension. *Am J Hypertens* 1989; **2**:259–61.

101. Timio M, Venanzi S, Lolli S, *et al.* "Non–dipper" hypertensive patients and progressive renal insufficiency: a 3–year longitudinal study. *Clin Nephrol* 1995; **43**:382–7.

102. Shimada K, Kawamoto A, Matsubayashi K, Nishinaga M, Kimura S, Ozawa T. Diurnal blood pressure variations and silent cerebrovascular damage in elderly patients with hypertension. *J Hypertens* 1992; **10**:875–8.

103. Ohkubo T, Imai Y, Tsuji I, *et al.* Relation between nocturnal decline in blood pressure and mortality. The Ohasama Study. *Am J Hypertens* 1997; **10**:1201–7.

104. Mancia G, Gamba PL, Omboni S, *et al.* Ambulatory blood pressure monitoring. *J Hypertens* 1996; **14** (Suppl):S61–6; discussion S66–8.

105. Mochizuki Y, Okutani M, Donfeng Y, *et al.* Limited reproducibility of circadian variation in blood pressure dippers and nondippers. *Am J Hypertens* 1998; **11**:403–9.

106. Ohkubo T, Imai Y, Tsuji I, *et al.* Reference values for 24–hour ambulatory blood pressure monitoring based on a prognostic criterion: the Ohasama Study. *Hypertension* 1998; **32**:255–9.

107. Pickering T. Recommendations for the use of home (self) and ambulatory blood pressure monitoring. American Society of Hypertension Ad-Hoc Panel. *Am J Hypertens* 1996; **9**:1–11.

108. Mar J, Pastor R, Abasolo R, Ruiz de Gauna R. Ambulatory blood pressure monitoring and diagnostic errors in hypertension: a Bayesian approach. *Med Decis Making* 1998; **18**:429–35.

109. Staessen JA, Byttebier G, Buntinx F, Celis H, O'Brien ET, Fagard R. Antihypertensive treatment based on conventional or ambulatory blood pressure measurement. A randomized controlled trial. Ambulatory Blood Pressure Monitoring and Treatment of Hypertension Investigators. *JAMA* 1997; **278**:1065–72.

110. Association for the Advancement of Medical Instrumentation. *American national standard for electronic or automated sphygmomanometers.* Arlington (VA): Association for the Advancement of Medical Instrumentation 1987.

111. O'Brien E, Petrie J, Littler W, *et al.* The British Hypertension Society protocol for the evaluation of automated and semi–automated blood pressure measuring devices with special reference to ambulatory systems. *J Hypertens* 1990; **8**:607–19.

Acknowledgements

We thank Ms Shirley Osborne for her invaluable assistance in collating the references for this chapter.

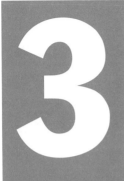

CHAPTER 3

How do cardiovascular risk factors affect whether we recommend therapy for hypertension?

Raj Padwal
Sharon E Straus
Finlay A McAlister

What blood pressure level is "hypertensive"?

What risk factors determine poor cardiovascular prognosis?

What tools help determine cardiovascular prognosis in individual patients, and how well do they work?

How do my patient and I decide whether treatment is worth considering?

Summary bottom lines

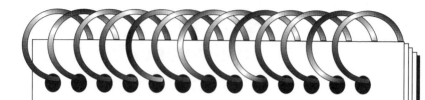

Patient Notes

Ms Athletic, age 45, fitness instructor

- Nonsmoker
- No family history of ischemic heart disease
- Healthy diet and activity lifestyle

Reason for visit

- Persistent average home BP 150/95 mm Hg for six months
- Work-up for secondary causes has been negative

Clinical findings

- Fasting glucose: 6.0 mmol/L
- Fasting lipid profile: total cholesterol 4.40 mmol/L;HDL 0.85 mmol/L;LDL 2.51 mmol/L
- Clinical examination, EKG, and urinalysis normal

Clinical question

- Should we initiate antihypertensive drug therapy in this middle-aged woman with low HDL cholesterol?

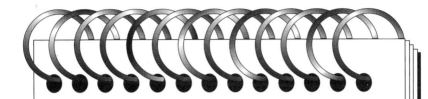

Patient Notes

Mr Reaven, age 45, sales executive

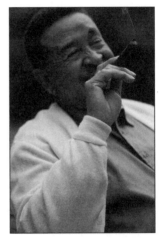

- Smoker
- Family history of premature myocardial infarction
- Trying diet and activity modification

Reason for visit

- Persistent average home BP 150/95 mm Hg for six months
- Work-up for secondary causes has been negative

Clinical findings

- Obese BMI 29
- Fasting glucose 8.0 mmol/L
- Fasting lipid profile: total cholesterol 7.14 mmol/L; HDL 1.85 mmol/L; LDL 4.95 mmol/L
- Clinical examination, EKG, and urinalysis normal

Clinical question

- Should we initiate antihypertensive therapy in this middle-aged man who smokes and has a family history of early cardiovascular disease?

What blood pressure level is "hypertensive"?

Blood pressure level and cardiovascular risk

Large population-based cohort studies consistently show continuous, strong, and graded relationships between blood pressure level and the subsequent occurrence of stroke,[1-13] myocardial infarction,[4-7,9,13-15] congestive heart failure,[4, 16] renal failure,[17] peripheral vascular disease,[4] cognitive decline,[18-21] and all-cause mortality.[7, 9, 11, 13, 22-27] (Pr: LI) There is no clear threshold value for blood pressure that accurately separates those who will and will not suffer future cardiovascular events (Figures 3.1 and 3.2).[6, 28] Relationships between blood pressure levels and cardiovascular disease are stronger for systolic than diastolic blood pressure levels and are consistent across multiple groups or types of patients.[15] Relationships are true for patients without known atherosclerotic disease as well as for those who have suffered a stroke or myocardial infarction.[3, 14]

Partial reversal of the cardiovascular risks that are associated with elevated blood pressure have been demonstrated in multiple high quality, long-term cohort studies (Pr: LI) and randomized clinical trials.[11, 29-36] (Tx: LI) Two important issues remain unclear: the exact level of blood pressure lowering that is associated with the greatest reduction in cardiovascular risk and whether the benefits of treatment are specifically tied to the level of blood pressure lowering (see Chapter 4).

Figure 3.1. Relationships between usual systolic blood pressure and risk of stroke, coronary heart disease, and all cause mortality as observed among men screened for the Multiple Risk Factor Intervention Trial(MRFIT).[5,22]

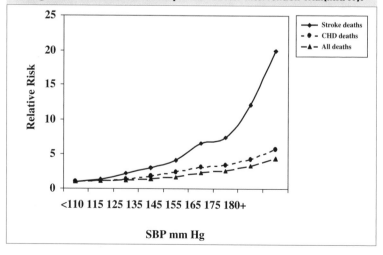

Figure 3.2. Relationships between usual diastolic blood pressure and risk of fatal and nonfatal stroke, fatal and nonfatal coronary heart disease (CHD), and all cause mortality

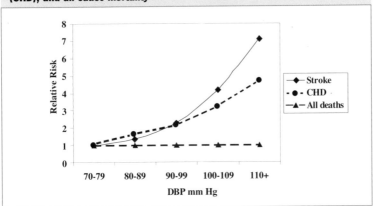

Stroke data were derived from a meta-analysis of 45 cohort studies (participant n=450 000);[4] Coronary heart disease data were derived from a meta-analysis of nine cohort studies (participant n=420 000);[6] all-cause mortality data were derived from the Chicago Heart Association Detection Project (participant n=21 220).[5]

Risk: absolute, relative, and attributable

Most population-based studies confirm that hypertension increases an individual's risk for various cardiovascular consequences approximately two- to threefold (Figure 3.3). The exact magnitude of the reported risks depends upon the follow-up duration and the blood pressure cut-off used to define hypertension in each study.[37]

The absolute risk to any individual for each cardiovascular consequence depends critically on the presence or absence of various metabolically linked risk factors and the presence or absence of target organ damage, particularly left ventricular hypertrophy.[4,15,28,38] For example, the following factors increase risk for coronary events in hypertensive individuals: elevated low-density lipoprotein (LDL) or total cholesterol, smoking, impaired glucose tolerance with or without diabetes mellitus, and reduced high-density lipoprotein (HDL) cholesterol.[4] Similarly, diabetes, valvular heart disease, myocardial infarction, and left ventricular hypertrophy are associated with increased risks for congestive heart failure in hypertensive individuals.[14]

The population attributable risk of hypertension for cardiovascular disease is tremendous. Hypertension causes approximately 35% of all atherosclerotic cardiovascular events,[4] 49% of all congestive heart failure,[16] and 24% of all premature deaths.[39]

Figure 3.3. Risk of atherosclerotic events in hypertensive compared to normotensive individuals.

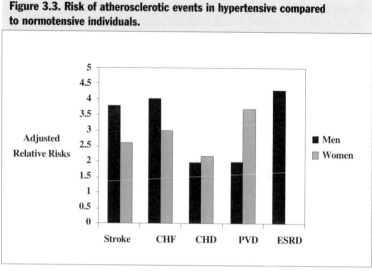

CHF	Congestive heart failure
CHD	Coronary heart disease
ESRD	End-stage renal disease
PVD	Peripheral vascular disease

Data were derived from 36-year follow-up of Framingham Study participants for all endpoints, except for ESRD data, which were derived from male Multiple Risk Factor Intervention Trial (MRFIT) participants.[4,17]

Defining the cut-point between normotension and hypertension

Blood pressure levels, like most physiological parameters, are normally distributed in the population. Neither the distribution of blood pressure in the population nor the relation between blood pressure and cardiovascular morbidity provides any justification for a rigid separation between normotension and hypertension.[40] Not surprisingly, there is substantial disagreement among consensus expert bodies on the definition of hypertension. Of the 27 national hypertension societies represented at the 17th World Hypertension League Council Conference in Montreal, Canada in 1997, 14 reported using a blood pressure level of 140/90 mm Hg to diagnose hypertension, and 13 used 160/95 mm Hg.[41] One definition, described by the Joint National Committee on Prevention, Detection, Evaluation, and Treatment of High Blood Pressure (JNC VI), is shown in Table 3.1.[42] This schema acknowledges a linear relationship between blood pressure level and cardiovascular risk and classifies patients into strata that are helpful in guiding whether antihypertensive treatment is warranted. Individuals in the high-normal stratum are at substantial risk for subsequently developing sustained hypertension with relative risks in excess of three for both men and women.[43](Pr: LI)

Table 3.1. Classification of blood pressure in adults.[42]

Category	Systolic blood pressure (mm Hg)	Diastolic blood pressure (mm Hg)
Optimal	< 120	< 80
Normal	< 130	< 85
High-normal	130 to 139	85 to 89
Hypertension		
Stage 1	140 to 159	90 to 99
Stage 2	160 to 179	100 to 109
Stage 3	≥ 180	≥ 110

When an individual's systolic and diastolic blood pressure fall into different categories, the higher category is used for classification.

What risk factors determine poor cardiovascular prognosis?

In the following section, we discuss multiple cardiovascular risk factors. We sort the risk factors into those that cannot be changed and those that can. Wherever possible, we summarize relative risks for cardiovascular morbidity and mortality, as well as the impact of therapy in reducing risks for those risk factors that are modifiable (Table 3.2). Causal relationships and reversals of risks with treatment are best established for hypertension and dyslipidemia. Evidence supporting independent causal effects for other cardiovascular risk factors is weaker for two reasons: they have been studied in highly selected populations with many confounding factors, and randomized controlled trials have not been conducted demonstrating clinical benefits when these risk factors are modified.

Nonmodifiable risk factors

Age

Cardiovascular risks clearly increase with increasing age.[4, 44–47](Pr: LI) A substantial proportion of this increased risk may be due to the increased prevalence of associated risk factors such as hypertension and diabetes; however, even after adjusting for other risk factors, older patients are at higher cardiovascular risk than their younger peers.

Gender

Cardiovascular disease is a leading cause of death in both men and women in Western countries. The incidence of myocardial infarction rises with age in both sexes, but is greater for men in each age category.[48](Pr: L1) The incidence in women is relatively low until the postmenopausal state is achieved.

Gender and interactions with other risk factors

Diabetes has a greater relative impact on cardiovascular disease incidence in women than in men (relative risk for female diabetics 3.7; relative risk for male diabetics 2.2).[44,49](Pr: L1) The relative risk of myocardial infarction was 1.6 in female compared to male smokers in a cohort study of over 24 000 individuals.[48,50](Pr: L1) Although diabetes and smoking are associated with smaller relative risks in men, the overall absolute risk in men is greater than in women.

Race

The incidence of cardiovascular disease varies amongst different races. It is not clear whether this variation is due to genetic polymorphisms or is a reflection of differences in socioeconomic status, access to healthcare resources, or cardiovascular risk factors. The third National Health and Nutrition Examination Survey shows highly significant differences in blood pressure, body mass index, physical activity, and prevalence of diabetes mellitus between ethnic groups in the United States, even after adjusting for educational differences.[51] Although some lower quality studies report that certain ethnic groups are at higher risk for cardiovascular events, most high quality evidence that adjusts for differences in baseline risk factors shows cardiovascular mortality rates are similar in Caucasians, African-Americans, Hispanics, and Asians.[5,52,53](Pr: L1) Likewise, the major cardiovascular risk factors, such as hypertension, dyslipidemia, smoking, and diabetes, exert similar relative risk increases across ethnic groups.[5, 52, 53]

Family history

A case-control study conducted within the framework of a large European trial showed that individuals who reported having relatives with premature coronary artery disease had substantially higher risks of myocardial infarctions than those without relatives with premature coronary heart disease. Relative risks were 2 in the instances of one affected relative and 3 in the instance of two or more affected relatives.[54](Pr: L3) Higher quality studies do not confirm the strength of this relationship; a large prospective cohort study shows a family history of premature coronary artery disease increases the relative risk of coronary heart disease by only 1.3.[55](Pr: L1)

Table 3.2. Magnitude of cardiovascular risk associated with risk factors that are potentially modifiable.

Risk factor	Range of relative risks from highest quality studies			Level of prognostic evidence
	Ischemic heart disease	Stroke	Total cardiovascular disease	
Hypertension	See text and Chapter 4			
Elevated LDL Decreased HDL	1.01 for each 1% increase in total cholesterol or LDL cholesterol or 1% reduction in HDL			1[45,56,57]
Elevated triglycerides			1.14 (men) to 1.37 (women) for each 1 mmol/L increase[58]	1
Elevated Lp(a)	1.61[59]	1.88[59]	1.44[59]	1
Smoking	1.2 to 2.24[38,44,46,50,55,57,60-62a]	1.5[47]		1
Diabetes mellitus	1.5 to 2.8 (men)[44,55,62,63]; 1.77 to 3.7 (women)[44,55,63]		2.61 (men) 2.24 (women)[63]	1
Sedentary lifestyle[b]			1.5 to 1.9[64,65]	1
Body weight and obesity[c]			1.7 (men; age under 50) 1.2 (men; age over 50) 2.1 (women; age under 50) 1.2(women; age over 50)[66]	1
Alcohol (moderate consumption)			0.6 to 0.7[67]	1
Left ventricular hypertrophy (EKG-LVH)	2.7 (men); 2.0 (women)[68]	1.8 (men); 4.0	3.1 (men); 3.3 (women)[69] (women)[68]	1
EKG-LVH (including strain)	3.0 to 4.0 (men); 2.3 to 4.6 (women)[44,68c]	1.7 to 5.8 (men); 3.3 to 6.2 (women)[44,68c]	5.84 men; (women)[69]	1
Microalbuminuria		See text		
Uric acid	NS[70]	1.5[71]	NS[70]	1 4
Plasma renin	3.8[72]	—	2.4[72]	2
Fibrinogen		2.3[73]	—	1
Homocysteine (for each 5μmol/L increase)	1.3[74]	1.5[75]	6.8[75]	1 3

NS: not significant; LP(a): lipoprotein (a)

[a]Risk varies according to amount and duration of exposure. See individual references for details.

[b]The numbers are referring to the least fit group compared to the fittest and second fittest group.

[c]Calculated from data in reference 66.

Potentially modifiable risk factors

Systolic and diastolic blood pressure

Systolic and diastolic blood pressures increase an average of 20/10 mm Hg from the ages of 35 to 60.[4] Thereafter, systolic blood pressure continues to rise with age due primarily to increased arterial stiffness, whereas diastolic blood pressure peaks at age 55 to 60 and then falls. The result is an increase in pulse pressure with increasing age. Systolic blood pressure is the most consistent and significant risk factor for cardiovascular disease and is an even stronger risk factor than diastolic blood pressure.[56, 76] It is also the most important risk factor for cerebrovascular disease in both men (relative risk 2.2) and women (relative risk 2.5).[44, 76] Further, isolated systolic hypertension is clearly associated with substantial risk of cardiovascular disease.[7, 9-11, 23, 25, 39] (Pr: LI)

Is this risk factor treatable?

Twelve-year follow-up data from the Multiple Risk Factor Intervention Trial (MRFIT) showed that a 7.5 mm Hg drop in diastolic blood pressure was associated with a 30% drop in cardiovascular disease mortality.[56] Pooled results of nine randomized trials involving approximately 43 000 patients followed for five to six years showed mean diastolic blood pressure in the treatment arm fell by an average of 5.7 mm Hg and mean systolic blood pressure fell 10.6 mm Hg.[77] The corresponding relative risk reduction in overall mortality was 11% (95% CI 2% to 19%) and in stroke-related mortality was 38% (95% CI 19% to 53%). There was also a trend towards a decrease in mortality from coronary heart disease by 8% and nonfatal myocardial infarction by 6%. Extrapolation of these data suggests that reducing diastolic blood pressure in a 35-year-old individual to 88 mm Hg could lead to increases in life spans of one to five years in men and one to six years in women, depending on pretreatment blood pressure levels.[78] (See Chapter 4 for more detail regarding treatment and its benefits.)

Pulse pressure

Traditionally, blood pressure has been determined by measuring peak systolic and diastolic pressure. An alternative approach is to view blood pressure as having two components: a steady state component represented by the mean arterial pressure and a dynamic, pulsatile component represented by the pulse pressure. Mean arterial pressure depends primarily on cardiac and peripheral vascular resistance, whereas ventricular ejection, arterial stiffness, and the timing of wave reflections determine pulse pressure.[79] Progressive increases in arterial stiffness with age cause earlier pulse-wave reflection. This leads to augmentation of the systolic blood pressure and a drop in the diastolic pressure so that pulse pressure increases with age.[80]

Several studies suggest that pulse pressure may be a stronger predictor of cardiovascular risk than either diastolic or systolic pressure in middle-aged and elderly patients.[81, 82](Pr: LI)

A recent meta-analysis examined the prognostic implications of widened pulse pressure in the elderly by combining data from three placebo-controlled trials.[79] Data were derived from 7882 predominantly Caucasian and Asian patients who were treated with several different antihypertensive agents. Adjusted analyses showed that a 10 mm Hg wider pulse pressure was associated with a 10% to 20% increased risk of death or cardiovascular disease (i.e., total mortality, cardiovascular mortality, coronary heart disease, and stroke). For a given level of systolic blood pressure, the cardiovascular risk increased with successively lower diastolic blood pressure values (Figure 3.4). Data from the large United States Hypertension Detection and Follow-up Program corroborated these findings; an increase in all-cause mortality by 11% was found for a pulse pressure increase of 10 mm Hg.[79, 83] In contrast, a similar rise of 10 mm Hg in systolic blood pressure and diastolic blood pressure resulted in increases in mortality of 8% and 5%, respectively.

Is this risk factor treatable?

Although there are antihypertensive agents that have varying effects on pulse pressure, no randomized trials have been conducted showing that agents with specific effects on pulse pressure lead to greater clinical benefits than do agents without such effects.

Lipid abnormalities

Elevations in serum total cholesterol concentration confer approximately a 1.9-fold increase in the risk of coronary disease in men and a 1.8-fold increase in women.[44](Pr: LI) An analysis of three international cohort studies shows up to 80% of the differences in mortality from ischemic heart disease between countries is explained by differences in serum cholesterol concentrations.[84] A strong, graded relationship between elevated cholesterol and coronary artery disease is seen with total cholesterol values greater than 4.65 mmol/L (180 mg/dL).[56] The protective effect of HDL cholesterol is at least as strong as the atherogenic effect of LDL, particularly in women.[48] Indeed, for every 1% decrease in HDL or increase in LDL, there is an associated 1% increase in coronary heart disease incidence in either sex.[57] (Pr: LI)

Is this risk factor treatable?

A recent meta-analysis of ten cohort studies suggested that a 0.6 mmol/L drop in total serum cholesterol concentration was associated with reductions in the incidence of ischemic heart disease of 54% at age 40, 39% at age 50, 27% at age 60, 20% at age 70, and 19% at age 80.[84](Pr: LI) There was no clear threshold level below which lowering serum cholesterol failed to decrease incidence of ischemic heart disease. Studies consistently found that it takes approximately five years to attain full benefit from treatment of cholesterol but that reductions in cardiovascular risk begin to appear relatively quickly: relative risk reductions 7% (95% CI 0% to 14%) after two years, 22% (95% CI 15% to 28%) from 2.1 to 5 years, and 25% (95% CI 15% to 35%) after five years.[84](Tx: LI)

A meta-analysis of five large statin trials showed that a 20% reduction in total cholesterol (28% reduction in LDL-C, 13% reduction in triglycerides, and a 5% increase in HDL-C) over five years translated into a 31% risk reduction in major coronary events (95% CI 26% to 36%) and a 21% reduction in all cause mortality (95% CI 14% to 28%).[85](Tx: LI) Relative risk reductions were similar in men and women, young and old, and in both primary and secondary prevention trials. Absolute risk reduction appeared greatest for patients with highest risk of cardiovascular disease.[86] Extrapolations showed that a reduction in total cholesterol from pretreatment levels of 240 mg/dL or greater to 200 mg/dL could increase life expectancy for 35-year-old individuals from two to four years in men and from two to six years in women, depending on baseline cholesterol levels.[78]

Figure 3.4. Risk associated with increasing systolic blood pressure at fixed levels of diastolic blood pressure (adapted with permission).[79]

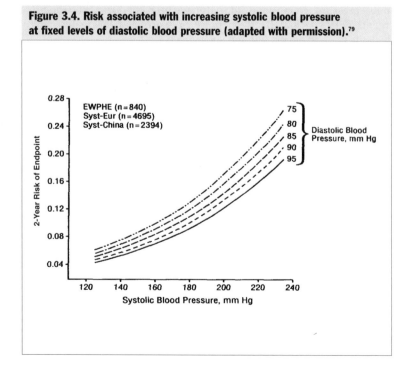

Triglycerides

Hypertriglyceridemia is a less well-established cardiovascular risk factor than elevated cholesterol and LDL values and low HDL values. One meta-analysis of 17 prospective cohort studies involving more than 57 000 patients found a relative risk of cardiovascular disease of 1.14 in men and 1.37 in women for each 1 mmol/L (88.6 mg/dL) increase in serum triglyceride levels.[58](Pr: LI) A secondary analysis of data from three large prospective studies (almost 16 000 subjects) found that triglyceride measurements did not improve heart disease risk estimation beyond that attainable using cholesterol measurements alone.[87]

Is this risk factor treatable?

Several trials suggest that reduced elevated triglyceride levels in patients with known coronary artery disease are associated with a reduction in clinically important cardiovascular disease.[88–90](Tx: 2B) We do not yet regard these trials as conclusive because trial participants had concomitant slight increases in HDL levels, which could partly explain the observed therapeutic benefits.

Lp(a)

Elevations of Lp(a), a heterogenous lipoprotein consisting of an LDL particle and a highly polymorphic apolipoprotein known as apolipoprotein(a), may predispose to cardiovascular disease via atherosclerotic and prothrombotic mechanisms.[91] While Level 4 cross-sectional and retrospective studies were the first to identify Lp(a) as a potential cardiovascular risk factor, nested case-control studies have shown conflicting results, with two of the four largest studies being negative.[59, 92–95](Pr: not classifiable) A large cohort study has shown that patients with sinking prebeta lipoprotein, a marker for elevated Lp(a), had a relative risk of 1.61 (95% CI 1.13 to 2.29) for coronary heart disease and 1.44 (95% CI 1.09 to 1.91) for total cardiovascular disease.[59](Pr: LI) Discrepant results between studies may be related to differences in sampling, storage techniques, standardization of assays, or definition of cardiovascular outcomes.[93] A cross-sectional study that investigated the association between Lp(a) and target-organ damage in an Italian population aged 35 to 65 years old suggested that Lp(a) levels were a better discriminator of the presence of target organ damage than systolic blood pressure, duration of hypertension or LDL-C.[96] Patients with a higher frequency of low-molecular-weight apo(a) isoforms exhibited more severe target organ damage.

Is this risk factor treatable?

We found no randomized controlled trials that investigated whether cardiovascular disease decreased with treatment of elevated Lp(a) levels.

Smoking

Smoking is a significant risk factor for cardiovascular disease. The risk is proportional to the number of cigarettes smoked and the depth of inhalation, and appears greater for women than men.[38, 47, 48, 50, 56, 97](Generally Pr: LI) The relative risk of myocardial infarction in smokers compared to nonsmokers is 1.4 (95% CI 1.3-1.6) for men and 2.2 (95% CI 1.9-2.7) for women.[50](Pr: LI) In a meta-analysis of 17 cohort studies, 14 case-control studies and 1 intervention trial, the relative risk of stroke associated with smoking was 1.5 (95% CI 1.4 to 1.6).[47](Pr: LI) Increased risk was particularly marked in younger individuals. Relative risks were 2.9 for people less than 55 years old, 1.8 for people aged 55 to 74 years old, and 1.1 for people older than 75 years of age. The overall relative risk in ex-smokers compared to nonsmokers was 1.2, and for those less than age 75 years old was 1.5. We found little data addressing the risks of pipe and cigar smoking, but one recent study suggested that such risks were intermediate between that of nonsmokers and cigarette smokers.[98](Pr: LI) For ischemic heart disease, a relative risk of 1.3 (95% CI 1.1 to 1.5) with a positive dose response relationship was reported.

Is this risk factor treatable?

Numerous studies show nicotine replacement and structured counseling both increase quit smoking rates.[99, 100](Tx: LI) We found no randomized trials that examined the effect of smoking cessation on clinical cardiovascular disease. Observational studies suggested that individuals with or without known coronary artery disease who stopped smoking seemed to gradually assume the cardiovascular risk profile of nonsmokers within one to three years, with the possible exception of the risk of peripheral vascular disease.[60,97,99,101](Pr: LI) In one large cohort of American men, reduction in smoking of ten cigarettes per day was associated with a 20% reduction in coronary and all-cause mortality.[102] (Pr: LI) Extrapolations suggest that reduction in the number of cigarettes smoked by 50% may add about 1.2 years to the life of a 35-year-old man and about 1.5 years to the life of a woman of similar age. Eliminating smoking altogether could increase life expectancy by about 2.3 years in men and 2.8 years in women.[78]

Diabetes

Diabetes is one of the strongest cardiovascular risk factors; associated age-adjusted risk ratios are about 2.2 for men and about 3.7 for women.[44](Pr: LI) Diabetes has greater relative impact in women compared to men for all types of cardiovascular disease, except congestive heart failure.[76] In general, mortality rates for coronary heart disease are three to seven times above baseline for diabetic women, compared to two to four times above baseline for diabetic men.[48] Diabetes often coexists with obesity, dyslipidemia, hypertension, and hyperuricemia. These coexisting risk factors have been given the label "Syndrome X"; patients with Syndrome X are particularly predisposed to atherosclerotic coronary artery disease.

Is this risk factor treatable?

Two large trials showed that blood glucose control in Type 1 and Type 2 diabetes delayed the development of microvascular diabetic complications, such as retinopathy, nephropathy and neuropathy.[103, 104] (Tx: LI) Neither trial showed improved glycemic control significantly decreased macrovascular disease, such as myocardial infarction. Analysis of the Framingham data suggested that diabetes exerted less impact on an individual's atherosclerotic risk than hypertension. Indeed, correction of hypertension is likely to provide more benefit in reducing macrovascular atherosclerotic disease than the control of diabetes.[55](Pr: LI)

Sedentary lifestyle

Many observational studies show associations between physical activity and lower incidence of coronary artery disease. However, they often fail to account for relationships between physical activity and higher HDL cholesterol levels, lower obesity rates, lower blood pressure levels, lower heart rates, and lower prevalence of smoking.[64,105] One study in middle-aged Norwegian men followed for 16 years has demonstrated that physical fitness was a graded and independent predictor of cardiovascular mortality.[65](Pr: LI) The adjusted-risk of cardiovascular mortality was directly related to the degree of physical fitness: relative risk was 0.41 (95% CI 0.20 to 0.84) in the most fit quartile, 0.45 (95% CI 0.22 to 0.92) in the second fittest group, and 0.59 (95% CI 0.28 to 1.22) in quartile 3, compared to the quartile with the lowest fitness ratings.[65] Similarly, a meta-analysis of five cohort studies found a 1.6-fold (95% CI 1.3 to 1.8) increase in coronary artery disease incidence among people with low activity levels compared to those with high activity levels.[64](Pr: LI)

Is this risk factor treatable?

Several randomized trials show that increasing regular physical activity among sedentary individuals is possible, though difficult to sustain. We found no randomized controlled trials that examined the effect of regular physical activity, compared to sedentary activity, on cardiovascular outcomes. In a prospective cohort study of 636 middle-aged Finnish men, those with higher physical activity levels lived an average of two years longer than those with lower levels ($p < 0.002$).(Pr: LI) However, the survival curves converged at the end of the 20-year follow-up period, which suggests that increased physical activity may not prolong the maximal achievable life span.[106]

Body weight and obesity

Increased body weight is one of the most prevalent cardiovascular risk factors in Western countries. Positive associations between body weight and incidence of cardiovascular disease are seen in both sexes after adjustment for other risk factors, though obesity is a more potent risk factor in women compared to men, and in younger compared to older people.[66](Pr: L1) Putative mechanisms for increased cardiovascular risk in obese people include associated higher prevalence of hypertension, dyslipidemia and diabetes, enhanced fibrinolytic activity and higher fibrinogen levels, and increased cardiac workload and intravascular volume.[107, 108] Whether lean body mass is associated with an increased risk of noncardiovascular mortality remains unclear, but observational data from people aged 60 years and older suggest an ideal body mass index of approximately 28 to 29 kg/m² for total mortality and approximately 26 to 27 kg/m² for cardiovascular mortality.[109, 110](Pr: L1)

Of the various anthropometric indices of central adiposity, attention has focused on the waist:hip ratio. Several cross-sectional studies have shown that elevated waist:hip ratios are associated with other risk factors such as hypertension and diabetes mellitus.[111–113] While multiple prospective studies have suggested that waist:hip ratios are a better predictor of stroke or coronary heart disease than measures of overall adiposity such as body mass index,[114–118] more recent studies suggest that the magnitude of this association may not be as strong as first thought given the frequent coexistence of elevated waist:hip ratio and other atherosclerotic risk factors. For example, a nested case-control study conducted within a prospective cohort study of almost 42 000 older women demonstrated that although waist:hip ratio was associated with the incidence of hypertension and stroke, this association was largely attenuated after adjusting for concomitant hypertension or diabetes mellitus (adjusted relative risk 1.3 [95% CI 0.8-2.1]).[119](Pr: L3)

Is this risk factor treatable?

Several randomized trials show that weight loss among obese individuals is possible, though difficult to sustain.[120](Tx: L1) We found no randomized controlled trials that examined the effect of weight loss, compared to either no change or weight gain, on clinical cardiovascular outcomes.

Alcohol

Observational studies consistently show inverse relationships between alcohol consumption and death from coronary heart disease.[121–123](Pr: L1, L2) For example, a large study of 490 000 Americans found the relative risk of cardiovascular death in subjects who consumed at least one drink per day compared to nondrinkers was 0.7 (95% CI 0.7-0.8) in men and 0.6 (95% CI 0.6-0.7) in women.[67](Pr: L1) Much of the beneficial effects of alcohol on coronary artery disease may be explained on the basis of improved HDL cholesterol profiles.[124] Although mild to moderate alcohol consumption appears to have protective cardiovascular effects, imbibing more than two drinks per day is associated with increased total mortality, due primarily to increased incidence of cancer, trauma and cirrhosis.[125]

Is this seemingly protective risk factor achievable?

We found no randomized controlled trials that examined the effects of consuming one to two alcoholic beverages compared to either more or less consumption on clinical cardiovascular outcomes.

Left ventricular hypertrophy

Studies using echocardiography, the most sensitive method of detection of left ventricular hypertrophy, show an estimated prevalence of 16% in hypertensive men and 23% in hypertensive women.[126] Although initially thought to represent only a compensatory mechanism from chronic pressure overload, left ventricular hypertrophy is now recognized as a strong predictor of future cardiovascular events, independent of blood pressure.[69, 126-129](Pr: LI) One large cohort study showed the age-adjusted odds ratio of cardiovascular disease for patients with left ventricular hypertrophy detected by electrocardiogram was 3.1 in men (95% CI 1.9 to 5.1) and 3.3 (95% CI 1.8 to 6.1) in women.[69](Pr: LI)

Compared to left ventricular hypertrophy, defined according to electrocardiogram voltage criteria alone, left ventricular hypertrophy with repolarization changes on electrocardiogram was associated with a 2.5-fold greater risk for cardiovascular disease.[126] Greater degrees of repolarization change were associated with greater increases in cardiovascular risk. Improvement in repolarization changes over time was associated with a strong trend towards a reduction in cardiovascular risk (odds ratio 0.5; 95% CI 0.2 to 1.01)[69] People experiencing serial declines in voltage on electrocardiogram are at lower risk for cardiovascular disease (men: odds ratio 0.5, 95% CI 0.3 to 0.8; women: odds ratio 0.6, 95% CI 0.3 to 1.04), and those with serial increases over time are at higher risk (men: odds ratio 1.9, 95% CI 1.1 to 3.0; women: odds ratio 1.6, 95% CI 0.9 to 2.8).[69]

Degree of cardiovascular risk also has been linked to abnormalities in left ventricular geometry including concentric remodeling (increased wall thickness with normal mass), eccentric hypertrophy (increased mass with normal thickness), and concentric hypertrophy (increased wall mass and thickness). While concentric hypertrophy appears to confer the greatest risk,[128, 130] it also is associated with the greatest mass, which suggests that left ventricular geometry does not add additional prognostic value.[4]

Is this risk factor treatable?

A meta-analysis of 39 high-quality randomized, double-blind trials showed that blood pressure reduction decreases in left ventricular mass. The magnitude of left ventricular hypertrophy regression was related to the degree of blood pressure reduction, the duration of therapy, and the left ventricular mass at baseline.[131](Tx: L1) After adjustment for different durations of treatment, there was some suggestion that drug class influenced the degree of left ventricular hypertrophy regression: ACE inhibitors decreased left ventricular mass index by 13.3% (95% CI 9.9% to 16.8%), calcium channel blockers by 9.3% (95% CI 5.5% to 13.1%), beta-blockers by 5.5% (95% CI 2.3% to 8.6%), and diuretics by 6.8% (95% CI 3.0% to 10.7%).[131] However, only 1200 and 189 patients received active and placebo treatment respectively and the mean duration of therapy was only 25 weeks.

We found no large randomized controlled trials that evaluated whether antihypertensive therapy that results in regression of left ventricular hypertrophy translates into a lower incidence of cardiovascular complications. We found two relatively small trials of short duration that reported encouraging preliminary results.[127,132](Tx: L2) Further evidence from larger randomized trials is needed to determine whether a decrease in left ventricular mass leads to a decrease in the risk of death and other clinically important outcomes.

Microalbuminuria

Microalbuminuria is defined as a urinary albumin excretion of 20 to 200 µg/min on a timed urine collection, or an excretion of 30 to 300 mg in a 24-hour period.[133] Using a mean of two to three measurements is suggested for diagnosis, because urinary albumin excretion is affected by multiple factors, including upright posture, higher blood pressure, exercise, obesity, smoking, and genetic or racial background.[133,134] Initial morning specimens tend to have the least variation.[133]

The reported prevalence of microalbuminuria among hypertensive individuals varies widely; a recent review cited prevalences of 10% to 37%.[134] Microalbuminuria reportedly has a higher prevalence in patients with the following conditions: more severe hypertension; more advanced target organ damage; no nocturnal drops in blood pressure (nondippers); higher renin levels; rises in blood pressure with increased salt intake (salt-sensitive), higher insulin levels and insulin resistance.[135-143] Traditional cardiovascular risk factors such as hyperlipidemia, obesity, and smoking also may increase urinary albumin excretion.[134-136, 138, 139] Therefore, it is not surprising that urinary albumin excretion rates are often increased in patients with cardiovascular disease.

There is conflicting evidence regarding whether microalbuminuria is an independent cardiovascular risk factor in patients with primary hypertension. Some preliminary studies suggest it adds independent predictive ability.[138,139,144](Pr: L2, L4) Another study suggests it predicts future cardiovascular mortality only among diabetic individuals and not in nondiabetic hypertensives.[145](Pr: L2) Whether microalbuminuria is predictive of eventual renal failure in patients with primary hypertension is also not definitively known.[142]

Is this risk factor treatable?

Preliminary evidence suggests that antihypertensive therapy causes regression of microalbuminuria, but studies done to date are small with relatively short durations of follow-up (weeks).[134] Reduction in arterial blood pressure, rather than intrinsic properties of specific antihypertensive agents, appears to be the major mechanism for regression of microalbuminuria. There is no convincing evidence for superiority of any particular class of antihypertensive medication.[134] We found no randomized controlled trials that investigated whether antihypertensive treatment specifically aimed at decreasing microalbuminuria results in improved long-term clinical outcomes.

Uric acid

As many as one-third of people with hypertension may have elevated uric acid levels, which may be an early indicator of hypertensive cardiorenal disease.[71] Hyperuricemia is associated with other coronary risk factors, such as obesity, impaired glucose tolerance, hypertension and hyperlipidemia. It also is seen in renal failure and may occur as a complication of treatment with beta-blockers or diuretics.

Whether hyperuricemia is an independent causative agent in the development of cardiovascular disease is unclear. At least two studies have shown continuous, graded relationships between serum uric acid levels and risk of cardiovascular disease (hazard ratio 1.2), myocardial infarction (relative risk 2.2), and stroke (relative risk 1.5).[71, 146](Pr: L2, L4) In contrast, a large cohort study showed no overall relationship between uric acid and risk of coronary heart disease or total cardiovascular disease after adjustment for associated risk factors.[70](Pr: L1) When potential confounding factors such as obesity and concomitant diuretic therapy were taken into account, serum uric acid was not an independent predictor of cardiovascular risk in several trials.[147, 148](Pr: L1)

Is this risk factor treatable?

We found no randomized controlled trials that investigated whether treatment specifically aimed at decreasing uric acid improves cardiovascular outcomes.

Plasma renin

Emerging evidence suggests that plasma renin may be an important cardiovascular risk factor. A large cohort study involving 2902 patients receiving antihypertensive treatment primarily with diuretics and beta-blockers found plasma renin was an independent risk factor for myocardial infarction (relative risk 3.8; 95% CI 1.7 to 8.4), total cardiovascular disease (relative risk 2.4; 95% CI 1.3 to 4.5) and all-cause mortality (relative risk 2.8; 95% CI 1.2 to 6.8).[72](Pr: L2) During a mean follow-up period of 3.6 years, a 2-unit increase in plasma renin levels was correlated with a 25% increase in myocardial infarction.

Is this risk factor treatable?

We found no randomized controlled trials that investigated whether treatment specifically aimed at decreasing renin levels improves cardiovascular outcomes.

Fibrinogen

Elevated fibrinogen often coexists with other cardiovascular risk factors such as smoking, diabetes and hypertension.[93,149] There is substantial individual variability in fibrinogen levels between patients and no single standardized assay, making it difficult to draw firm conclusions across different studies. One large American cohort study found fibrinogen was an independent risk factor for cardiovascular disease.[44](Pr: L1) In a large Scottish survey of 10 359 men and women aged 40 to 59 years, plasma fibrinogen levels were positively associated with angina, myocardial infarction, and a family history of premature heart disease, hypertension, diabetes, and intermittent claudication.[149](Pr: L4) A meta-analysis of six studies showed that the odds ratio was 2.3 (95% CI 1.9 to 2.8) for coronary disease for the highest compared with the lowest tertile of fibrinogen level.[73](Pr: L1)

Is this risk factor treatable?

We found no large randomized controlled trials that investigated whether treatment specifically aimed at decreasing fibrinogen levels results in improved clinical cardiovascular outcomes. However, preliminary evidence, from a secondary analysis of patients in a randomized trial designed to test the impact of fibrates in patients with known coronary atherosclerosis and abnormal lipid profiles, suggests that reduction of elevated fibrinogen levels may be associated with reduction in fatal/nonfatal myocardial infarction, stroke, and death.[150] (Tx: L4) Although the authors reported relative risk reductions for stroke of nearly two-thirds in that subgroup of patients with both the highest tertile of baseline fibrinogens and the highest tertile of fibrinogen lowering, the analysis was seriously flawed. The subgroup and its comparators were developed based on post-hoc analysis of data, and results were presented without adjusting for treatment allocation or differences in lipid profile at baseline and during the trial.[150]

Homocysteine

Observational studies suggest that moderate levels of homocysteine elevation are associated with increased risk of cardiovascular disease.[74, 75, 151, 152](Pr: L2, L3) Specifically, a meta-analysis of 27 studies suggested an association between homocysteine and atherosclerotic vascular disease.[75] (L3, L4) Each 5 µmol/L increase in basal total plasma homocysteine levels was associated with an odds ratio for coronary artery disease of 1.6 (95% CI 1.4 to 1.7) in men and 1.8 (95% CI 1.3 to1.9) in women. The summary odds ratios for the same increment in baseline total homocysteine levels were 1.5 (95% CI 2.0 to 3.0) for cerebrovascular disease and 6.8 (95 % CI 2.9 to 15.8) for peripheral vascular disease. The authors estimated that 10% of the population's coronary artery disease risk may be attributable to elevated homocysteine levels.[75] However, higher quality studies in the meta-analysis reported weaker associations between homocysteine and cardiovascular risk. [74,151](Pr: L2) A more recent systematic review summarized the results of the five highest quality case-control studies, in which data was collected prospectively and differences in age, gender, and other cardiovascular risk factors were controlled for in adjusted analyses. These authors found a less convincing association with coronary heart disease (odds ratio of 1.3 [95% CI 1.1-1.5] for each 5 µmol/L increase in homocysteine levels) and substantial heterogeneity between the published studies.[74](Pr: L1)

Is this risk factor treatable?

We found no completed randomized controlled trials that investigated whether treatment specifically aimed at decreasing homocysteine levels results in improved cardiovascular outcomes, but several such trials are currently underway.[152]

Infectious agents and low-grade inflammation

Emerging evidence suggests that coronary heart disease is probably not associated with infectious agents, such as *Chlamydia pneumoniae* but that it probably is associated with some low-grade inflammatory processes.[153] An early small case-control study reported an association between elevated titers of *Chlamydia pneumoniae* and stroke (relative risk 8.6; 95% CI 1.07 to 68.9), as well as cardiac events (relative risk 2.7; 95% CI 1.04 to 7.0).[154](Pr: L3) Subsequently, a nested case-control study within a large British prospective study of professional men found no material association between *Chlamydia pneumoniae* and ischemic heart disease.[155] A meta-analysis of all 15 prospective studies evaluating serological evidence of *Chlamydia pneumoniae* infection excluded any strong association between those titres and incident coronary heart disease.[156] (Pr: L1) A meta-analysis of 14 prospective studies found people with the highest tertiles of C-reactive protein, a marker of low grade inflammation, had more coronary heart disease than those in the bottom tertile (summary risk ratio 1.9, 95% CI 1.5 to 2.3).[157](Pr: Ll) However, it is still unclear whether C-reactive protein is an independent risk factor for atherosclerotic disease, given the lack of direct evidence that C-reactive protein contributes to vascular damage and the marked reduction in putative effect size that is seen after adjustment for baseline differences in confounders.[157]

Is this risk factor treatable?

We found no randomized controlled trials that investigated whether treatment specifically aimed at infectious agents improves cardio-vascular outcomes.

Other risk factors

Several additional potential "risk" factors for cardiovascular disease are being studied, including HDL3, apolipoprotein B, albumin, von Willebrand factor, factor VIII activity, leukocyte count, and high-risk genotypes, such as an angiotensin genotype.[158] As of June 2000, we found no large high-quality prospective studies that had established the independent significance of these factors.

What tools help determine cardiovascular prognosis in individual patients, and how well do they work?

As already discussed, blood pressure level is only one of many risk factors for cardiovascular disease. The risk of cardiovascular morbidity or mortality in individuals with mild hypertension depends more on their constellation of risk factors than their actual blood pressure reading.[4,38,55,159-164](Pr: Ll) In order to estimate the prognosis for individual patients, we need to estimate their absolute risk for cardiovascular disease and the efficacy of treatment.[28,159] For example, a 40-year-old man with a blood pressure of 160/95 mm Hg who is otherwise healthy and does not smoke has a 10-year risk of less than 10% of suffering a cardiovascular event such as stroke, myocardial infarction, or coronary death. On the other hand, a 40-year-old man with the same blood pressure who smokes, is obese, and has dyslipidemia has a 10-year risk of approximately 20 to 40%.[165] We describe below numerous methods that can be used to estimate such individual absolute cardiovascular risks.

Framingham risk equations

These equations were derived from over 5300 individuals aged 30 to 74 years from both the original and offspring Framingham studies. They are regression equations for the prediction of cardiovascular disease defined as coronary disease, congestive heart failure, or stroke.[55, 166, 167] These clinical prediction guides have been validated in data sets other than those from which they were derived and, as such, represent Level 1 prognostic information. Earlier iterations of these equations included multivariate-adjusted scores for various atherosclerotic risk factors: age, sex, total cholesterol, HDL cholesterol, systolic blood pressure, cigarette smoking, diabetes, and left ventricular hypertrophy on electro-cardiogram.[168] A refinement of these equations that incorporated LDL-cholesterol and diastolic blood pressure and removed left ventricular hypertrophy on electrocardiogram is shown in Appendix 1. This refinement permits estimation of an individual patient's risk of coronary heart disease defined as angina pectoris, myocardial infarction, coronary insufficiency or coronary heart disease death.[55]

Use of these risk prediction equations is best illustrated by considering our two patients, Ms Athletic and Mr Reaven. Working through risk assessment for women with Ms Athletic reveals that her point total is 10 points, which corresponds to an estimated 10-year coronary heart disease risk of 10%. The average risk of a 45-year-old female is 5% over 10 years. Dividing Ms Athletic's risk by the average risk reveals that her relative risk is 2.0. On the other hand, working through risk assessment for men for our second patient, Mr Reaven, reveals a point total of 8 points, which corresponds to an estimated 10-year coronary heart disease risk of 16%. The average risk for a 45-year-old male is 11% over 10 years. Dividing Mr Reaven's risk by the average risk reveals that his relative risk is 1.5. Thus, Ms Athletic is at higher relative risk than Mr. Reaven, but lower absolute risk. We consider the merits of basing treatment decision on absolute rather than relative risk later in this chapter.

Although the Framingham investigators have urged caution in extrapolating from the Framingham cohort of predominantly Caucasian, middle-class Americans recruited from an area near Boston to other populations, the risk equations have been shown to be reasonably accurate when applied to other populations in Northern Europe and other centers in the United States.[169–172] Thus, numerous international guidelines[165, 173–175] advise formal risk estimation using simplified versions of the Framingham risk equations and specify absolute risk treatment thresholds. However, the Framingham equations appear to overestimate coronary risk in French, Puerto Rican, and Hawaiian populations, and another North American-derived risk function overestimated risk in Japanese and southern European cohorts.[176–178] The Framingham risk equations also have been criticized for not including several

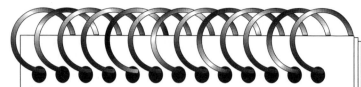

Patient Notes: What is Ms Athletic's relative risk?

Age, 45	3 pts
Nonsmoker	0 pts
Nondiabetic	0 pts
Total cholesterol 4.40 mmol/L	0 pts
HDL 0.83 mmol/L	5 pts
BP 150/95	2 pts
Point total	10 pts
10-year risk of CV disease	10%

What does this mean?

Average risk of a 45-year-old female is 5% over 10 years. Dividing Ms Athletic's risk by the average risk reveals that her relative risk is 2.0 for suffering a cardiovascular event in the next 10 years.

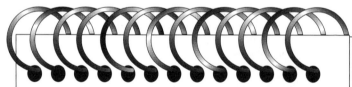

Patient Notes: What is Mr Reaven's relative risk?

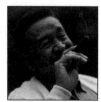

Age, 45	2 pts
Smoker	2 pts
Diabetic	2 pts
Total cholesterol 7.14 mmol/L	2 pts
HDL 1.85 mmol/L	-2 pts
BP 150/95	2 pts
Point total	8 pts
10-year risk of CV disease	16%

What does this mean?

Average risk of a 45-year-old male is 11% over 10 years. Dividing Mr Reaven's risk by the average risk reveals that his relative risk is 1.5 for suffering a cardiovascular event in the next 10 years.

atherosclerotic risk factors such as family history, sedentary lifestyle, and obesity which, at least on univariate analysis, appear to weakly predict risk. However, it could be argued that these risk factors are likely minor players and are not strongly and independently related to risk in multivariate analyses.

Cardiovascular Disease Life Expectancy Model

This is a Markov Model that was developed using data from the Lipid Research Clinics Follow-up Cohort of approximately 3700 people aged 35 to 74 years, the Canadian Heart Health Survey, and Canadian life tables. It incorporates age, gender, mean blood pressure, total and HDL cholesterol levels, and the presence or absence of diabetes mellitus, smoking, or cardiovascular disease in calculating absolute risk.[179] As this model has been validated in data sets other than those from which it was derived, it also represents a Level 1 prognostic clinical prediction guide. It holds several advantages over the Framingham risk equations. First, it provides a single estimate for the risk of coronary events, death, or strokes in any one individual. There are two separate Framingham equations for coronary events and strokes, and no means to combine the two to predict the risk of stroke and/or coronary events in the same patient. Second, this model was derived from a cohort of individuals with and without overt coronary heart disease and thus can be used to predict the potential benefits of risk factor modification both before and after the development of symptomatic coronary disease. The Framingham equations were derived only in people without symptomatic coronary disease. Third, this model has been validated using data from both primary and secondary prevention trials and thus can be used to estimate the effectiveness and cost-effectiveness of various risk factor modifications in a wide range of patients. The major disadvantage of this model is that it requires access to the original formulae and is not yet available in a simple chart form such as Appendices 1 and 2.

The Dundee Coronary Risk Disk

This risk equation was derived from approximately 5200 men aged 40 to 59 years attending various general practices in the United Kingdom.[180] The equation incorporates information on total cholesterol, systolic blood pressure, and smoking. It provides an estimate of an individual's relative risk for coronary mortality versus their age and sex peer group. It was derived solely in men and has not been independently validated in women. Although it has been validated in a second cohort of British men, information regarding its generalizability is limited and its predictive abilities correlate only modestly with the Framingham estimates (correlation coefficient $r = 0.68$).[169]

The PROCAM Risk Function

This risk equation was derived in 4400 employees aged 40 to 65 years old in Munster, Germany. It includes age, total and HDL cholesterol, systolic blood pressure, smoking, family history, diabetes, and anginal symptoms.[181] Although there is a moderate correlation between PROCAM risk estimates and those derived from the Framingham equation (r=0.82, p<0.0001), it has not been independently validated in women and its generalizability to other populations is unknown.[169]

The British Regional Heart Study Risk Function

This risk equation was derived in 7700 British male factory workers aged 40 to 59 years. It incorporates total cholesterol, mean blood pressure, smoking, diabetes, symptomatic ischemic heart disease, and family history.[182] It has never been validated in an independent test set, cannot be used to predict coronary risk in women, and has been found to systematically underestimate risk when compared to all other risk functions.[169]

Advantages and disadvantages of using estimates of absolute risk to guide treatment

In the hope that antihypertensive drug therapy will be most efficient and effective if directed at those who, by virtue of their constellation of risk factors or evidence of preclinical vascular disease, are likely to have a heart attack or stroke, numerous hypertension guidelines advocate explicit consideration of an individual patient's absolute risk of subsequent cardiovascular disease in the decision to initiate therapy.[28,159] These "risk-based" guidelines have several advantages over traditional guidelines. They inform patient and provider decision-making by explicitly quantifying the magnitude of expected benefits and harms of treatment. As individual treatment decisions are based on the potential of the individual to benefit from an intervention, the benefit to harm ratio is maximized for each patient. Preliminary evidence suggests that physicians do implicitly stratify their patients by risk category in deciding whether to initiate antihypertensive therapy.[183] It seems reasonable to hypothesize that adherence rates and patient outcomes may be better with risk-based guidelines than those demonstrated with traditional hypertension guidelines, particularly since consideration of "the risk to health without therapy" plays an important role in clinical decision-making.[184, 185] Physicians tend to view therapies that confer large absolute benefits more favorably than those associated with large relative risk reductions but more modest absolute benefits.[186]

We acknowledge several shortcomings to the use of risk-based guidelines. The primary problem lies in the fact that these guidelines currently depend on risk-prediction equations, such as the Framingham equations discussed above, which have some weaknesses, may not be generalizable to all populations, and are incapable of rapidly incorporating emerging evidence on newly-appreciated risk factors. A second problem with risk-based guidelines, at least as currently envisioned, is that they concentrate on risk over a finite period of time (such as five or ten years) rather than the lifetime risk from hypertension. This may be a significant flaw because the calculation of benefit on the basis of short-term randomized clinical trials might seriously underestimate the long-term benefits from antihypertensive therapy.[187] Similarly, these guidelines tend to focus on endpoints, such as stroke or myocardial infarction, and do not include other important consequences of hypertension, such as heart failure, renal failure, or peripheral vascular disease. Finally, the use of absolute risk treatment thresholds raises troubling ethical questions, which require explicit acknowledgement and debate. They favor treatment of the elderly at the expense of younger patients, men rather than women, and smokers over nonsmokers.[159]

 # How do my patient and I decide whether treatment is worth considering?

Absolute risk profiles and risk-based guidelines do not solve the problem of setting treatment thresholds for guideline developers or for individual clinicians treating individual patients. Guidelines often specify different treatment thresholds for the patient with uncomplicated, mild essential hypertension (for example, 140 to 159/90 to 99 mm Hg), and patients and clinicians often vary in their treatment preferences.[188, 189] As the majority of hypertensive individuals have blood pressures in the range mentioned above, discrepancies in treatment thresholds have important implications (Table 3.3).[159]

The process by which treatment thresholds are chosen is rarely explicit. As there is a direct relationship between diastolic and systolic blood pressure and the risk of cardiovascular endpoints, the clinical trial literature does not illuminate a specific threshold separating those who will derive benefit from therapy from those who will be harmed. Thus, it seems reasonable to incorporate the opinions of patients and front-line clinicians both when setting treatment thresholds and when discussing with an individual patient whether or not to start treatment.[63, 190, 191]

Patient or physician preferences can be elicited by determining the smallest amount of benefit which they perceive as outweighing the side effects, cost, and inconvenience of antihypertensive therapy: their minimal clinically important difference (MCID).[192] Probability trade-off tools originally developed for cancer patients can be used to elicit MCIDs. Clinicians present background information on the disease, treatment options, and potential outcomes, and then ask patients to choose between not taking therapy (given their baseline risk of an adverse outcome) or taking therapy (given a reduced risk of the adverse outcome but also incurring the inconvenience, side effects, and costs associated with that therapy[188]). For example, patients could be presented the following: (a) their baseline risk for cardiovascular events; (b) the potential benefits of treatment expressed as absolute risk reductions; and (c) an estimate of the frequency and type of adverse effects, including inconvenience and costs. After assessing the patient's understanding of such pros and cons of treatment, their preferences are ascertained.

Table 3.3. Implications of different treatment thresholds for patients with uncomplicated essential hypertension.[159,191]

Diastolic blood pressure	90 mm Hg	95 mm Hg	100 mm Hg
Risk of cardiovascular event[a]			
In 5 years	2%	5%	10%
In 20 years	15%	30%	50%
NNT to prevent one cardiovascular event[b]			
In 5 years	200	80	40
In 20 years	27	13	8
Percentage of population eligible for treatment	25	14	8

NNT   number needed to treat
[a]Cardiovascular risks were calculated from the Cardiovascular Disease Life Expectancy Model, assuming the patient was 45 years old and had the average risk factor profile seen in Canadian hypertensives (risks for men and women averaged).[179]
[b]Assuming relative risk reductions with treatment of 25% for any cardiovascular event.[33,34,191]

We illustrate joint informed decision-making by returning to Ms Athletic and Mr Reaven. We inform Ms Athletic that her baseline risk of coronary events (calculated from the Framingham equation as outlined above) is 10% in the next 10 years. As the relative risk reductions in cardiovascular events seen with antihypertensive treatment are approximately 25% in all subgroups,[33] we are able to tell Ms Athletic that taking antihypertensive therapy to lower her blood pressure will reduce her risk to 7.5% (or lower, given the underestimation of benefit in hypertension trials discussed above). Her costs will probably include having to take one or two pills a day, costing $10 to 40 per month. The risk of adverse effects including their exact frequency and nature will vary depending on which antihypertensive drug is chosen. As Ms Athletic values her active lifestyle and is reluctant to take medication (she wishes to avoid any perception that she is "ill"), she decides this benefit is insufficient to accept treatment. However, she does agree to modify her lifestyle and consume increased fish oils in an effort to raise her serum HDL cholesterol, the major risk factor driving her increased risk as outlined above.

On the other hand, after we inform Mr Reaven of his baseline risk of coronary events (calculated as 16% in the next 10 years using the Framingham equation), the potential to reduce this by 4% with the same costs, inconvenience, and potential adverse effects faced by Ms Athletic, he decides to accept long-term treatment. In addition, he agrees to attend a quit-smoking counseling program.

In the case of the policy maker setting treatment thresholds for guidelines, a sample of patients and clinicians can be presented with various scenarios outlining different baseline risks and the hypothetical benefits from therapy can be varied until the mean or median treatment thresholds of both groups are apparent. This approach has been piloted in Canadian and British settings and the preliminary data suggest that guidelines which set treatment thresholds on the basis of physician or expert opinion do not accurately reflect the preferences of hypertensive individuals.[188, 189] Coupled with evidence that patients want to be more involved in decision-making,[193, 194] there is a clear need for patient decision aids and attention to patient preferences when considering the initiation of antihypertensive therapy for the prevention of cardiovascular disease.

Summary bottom lines

- Advise patients that there is a continuous, strong, and graded relationship between blood pressure level and the incidence of cardiovascular disease. No clear threshold value of blood pressure separates those hypertensive patients who will suffer future cardiovascular events from those who will not. (Level 1 evidence)

- Advise patients that their individual risk of cardiovascular disease depends on their blood pressure level, coexistent risk factors, and whether or not they have hypertensive target organ damage. (Level 1 evidence)

- Inform patients that numerous factors have been shown to increase cardiovascular risk. The two risk factors most strongly tied to poor prognosis are hypertension and lipid abnormalities. Other risk factors include: male gender, family history of premature cardiac disease, older age, smoking, diabetes mellitus, sedentary lifestyle, obesity (particularly central adiposity), left ventricular hypertrophy, microalbuminuria, elevations of plasma uric acid, renin, fibrinogen, homocysteine, and markers of low grade inflammation such as C-reactive protein. (Level 1 and 2 evidence)

- Consider using validated models to estimate a patient's absolute risk for cardiovascular disease and the efficacy of treatment. The most widely

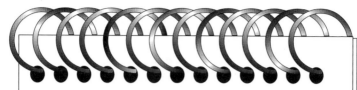

Patient Notes

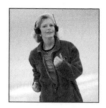

Decision for Ms Athletic

- 10-year cardiovascular risk: 10%

Benefit and cost of treatment

- Reduce risk from 10% to 7.5% in next 10 years.
- One or two pills a day, costing $10-$40 per month, with risk of adverse effects.

Informed decision

She decides benefit does not outweigh risks, and chooses no medication. But she agrees to modify her lifestyle and to consume more fish oils to raise her HDL.

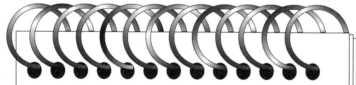

Patient Notes

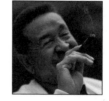

Decision for Mr Reaven

- 10-year cardiovascular risk: 16%

Benefit and cost of treatment

- Reduce risk from 16% to 12% in next 10 years.
- One or two pills a day, costing $10-$40 per month, with risk of adverse effects.

Informed decision

He decides benefit does outweigh risks, and chooses to take antihypertensive medication and attend a quit-smoking counseling program.

used are the Framingham Risk Prediction Equations. Considering risk in the decision to initiate therapy explicitly quantifies the magnitude of expected benefits and harms of treatment. (Consensus opinion)

We identified information for this chapter by searching MEDLINE from 1966 to 2000. We specifically searched for English language, human literature relevant to hypertension and cardiovascular risk. We screened approximately 2000 titles and/or abstracts to help identify the highest quality relevant information to include in this chapter.

 References

1. Prospective Studies Collaboration. Cholesterol, diastolic blood pressure, and stroke: 13 000 strokes in 450 000 people in 45 prospective cohorts. *Lancet* 1995; **346**:1647-53.

2. Disease Collaborative Research Group. Blood pressure, cholesterol, and stroke in eastern Asia. Eastern Stroke and Coronary Heart. *Lancet* 1998; **352**:1801-7.

3. Rodgers A, MacMahon S, Gamble G, Slattery J, Sandercock P, Warlow C. Blood pressure and risk of stroke in patients with cerebrovascular disease. The United Kingdom Transient Ischaemic Attack Collaborative Group. *BMJ* 1996; **313**:147.

4. Kannel WB. Blood pressure as a cardiovascular risk factor: prevention and treatment. *JAMA* 1996; **275**:1571-6.

5. Stamler J, Stamler R, Neaton JD. Blood pressure, systolic and diastolic, and cardiovascular risks. US population data. *Arch Intern Med* 1993; **153**:598-615.

6. MacMahon S, Peto R, Cutler J, *et al.* Blood pressure, stroke, and coronary heart disease. Part 1: Prolonged differences in blood pressure: prospective observational studies corrected for the regression dilution bias. *Lancet* 1990; **335**:765-74.

7. Antikainen R, Jousilahti P, Tuomilehto J. Systolic blood pressure, isolated systolic hypertension and risk of coronary heart disease, strokes, cardiovascular disease and all-cause mortality in the middle-aged population. *J Hypertens* 1998; **16**:577-83.

8. He J, Klag MJ, Wu Z, Whelton PK. Stroke in the People's Republic of China. II. Meta-analysis of hypertension and risk of stroke. *Stroke* 1995; **26**:2228-32.

9. O'Donnell CJ, Ridker PM, Glynn RJ, *et al.* Hypertension and borderline isolated systolic hypertension increase risks of cardiovascular disease and mortality in male physicians. *Circulation* 1997; **95**:1132-7.

10. Nielsen WB, Vestbo J, Jensen GB. Isolated systolic hypertension as a major risk factor for stroke and myocardial infarction and an unexploited source of cardiovascular prevention: a prospective population-based study. *J Hum Hypertens* 1995; **9**:175-80.

11. Staessen JA, Gasowski J, Wang JG, *et al.* Risks of untreated and treated isolated systolic hypertension in the elderly: meta-analysis of outcome trials. *Lancet* 2000; **355**:865-72.

12. Nielsen WB, Lindenstrom E, Vestbo J, Jensen GB. Is diastolic hypertension an independent risk factor for stroke in the presence of normal systolic blood pressure in the middle-aged and elderly? *Am J Hypertens* 1997; **10**:634-9.

13. Selmer R. Blood pressure and twenty-year mortality in the city of Bergen, Norway. *Am J Epidemiol* 1992; **136**:428-40.

14. Flack JM, Neaton J, Grimm R Jr, *et al.* Blood pressure and mortality among men with prior myocardial infarction. Multiple Risk Factor Intervention Trial Research Group. *Circulation* 1995; **92**:2437-45.

15. Van Den Hoogen PC, Feskens EJ, Nagelkerke NJ, Menotti A, Nissinen A, Kromhout D. The relation between blood pressure and mortality due to coronary heart disease among men in different parts of the world. Seven Countries Study Research Group. *N Engl J Med* 2000; **342**:1-8.

16. Levy D, Larson MG, Vasan RS, Kannel WB, Ho KK. The progression from hypertension to congestive heart failure. *JAMA* 1996; **275**:1557-62.

17. Klag MJ, Whelton PK, Randall BL, *et al.* Blood pressure and end-stage renal disease in men. *N Engl J Med* 1996; **334**:13-18.

18. Kilander L, Nyman H, Boberg M, Hansson L, Lithell H. Hypertension is related to cognitive impairment: a 20-year follow-up of 999 men. *Hypertension* 1998; **31**:780-6.

19. Skoog I, Lernfelt B, Landahl S, *et al.* 15-year longitudinal study of blood pressure and dementia. *Lancet* 1996; **347**:1141-5.

20. Barash PG. Preoperative evaluation of the cardiac patient for noncardiac surgery. *Can J Anaesth* 1991; **38**:R134-44.

21. Elias MF, Wolf PA, D'Agostino RB, Cobb J, White LR. Untreated blood pressure level is inversely related to cognitive functioning: the Framingham Study. *Am J Epidemiol* 1993; **138**:353-64.

22. Stamler J. Blood pressure and high blood pressure. Aspects of risk. *Hypertension* 1991; **18**:I95-107.

23. Port S, Demer L, Jennrich R, Walter D, Garfinkel A. Systolic blood pressure and mortality. *Lancet* 2000; **355**:175-80.

24. Glynn RJ, Field TS, Rosner B, Hebert PR, Taylor JO, Hennekens CH. Evidence for a positive linear relation between blood pressure and mortality in elderly people. *Lancet* 1995; **345**:825-9.

25. Weijenberg MP, Feskens EJ, Kromhout D. Blood pressure and isolated systolic hypertension and the risk of coronary heart disease and mortality in elderly men (the Zutphen Elderly Study). *J Hypertens* 1996; **14**:1159-66.

26. Kaufman JS, Rotimi CN, Brieger WR, *et al.* The mortality risk associated with hypertension: preliminary results of a prospective study in rural Nigeria. *J Hum Hypertens* 1996; **10**:461-4.

27. Fletcher AE, Bradley IC, Broxton JS, *et al.* Survival of hypertensive subjects identified on screening: results for sustained and unsustained diastolic hypertension. *Eur Heart J* 1992; **13**:1595-601.

28. Alderman MH. Blood pressure management: individualized treatment based on absolute risk and the potential for benefit. *Ann Intern Med* 1993; **119**:329-35.

29. Hunink MG, Goldman L, Tosteson AN, *et al.* The recent decline in mortality from coronary heart disease, 1980-1990. The effect of secular trends in risk factors and treatment. *JAMA* 1997; **277**:535-42.

30. Mosterd A, D'Agostino RB, Silbershatz H, *et al.* Trends in the prevalence of hypertension, antihypertensive therapy, and left ventricular hypertrophy from 1950 to 1989. *N Engl J Med* 1999; **340**:1221-7.

31. Sytkowski PA, D'Agostino RB, Belanger AJ, Kannel WB. Secular trends in long-term sustained hypertension, long-term treatment, and cardiovascular mortality. The Framingham Heart Study 1950 to 1990. *Circulation* 1996; **93**:697-703.

32. Forette F, Seux ML, Staessen JA, *et al.* Prevention of dementia in randomised double-blind placebo-controlled Systolic Hypertension in Europe (Syst-Eur) trial. *Lancet* 1998; **352**:1347-51.

33. Gueyffier F, Boutitie F, Boissel JP, *et al.* Effect of antihypertensive drug treatment on cardiovascular outcomes in women and men. A meta-analysis of individual patient data from randomized, controlled trials. The INDANA Investigators. *Ann Intern Med* 1997; **126**:761-7.

34. Collins R, Peto R, MacMahon S, *et al.* Blood pressure, stroke, and coronary heart disease. Part 2: Short-term reductions in blood pressure: overview of randomised drug trials in their epidemiological context. *Lancet* 1990; **335**:827-38.

35. MacMahon S, Rodgers A. Blood pressure, antihypertensive treatment and stroke risk. *J Hypertens* 1994; **12**(Suppl):S5-14.

36. Kostis JB, Davis BR, Cutler J, *et al.* Prevention of heart failure by antihypertensive drug treatment in older persons with isolated systolic hypertension. SHEP Cooperative Research Group. *JAMA* 1997; **278**:212-16.

37. Marang-Van De Mheen PJ, Gunning-Schepers LJ. Variation between studies in reported relative risks associated with hypertension: time trends and other explanatory variables. *Am J Public Health* 1998; **88**:618-22.

38. Lowe LP, Greenland P, Ruth KJ, Dyer AR, Stamler R, Stamler J. Impact of major cardiovascular disease risk factors, particularly in combination, on 22-year mortality in women and men. *Arch Intern Med* 1998; **158**:2007-14.

39. O'Donnell CJ, Kannel WB. Cardiovascular risks of hypertension: lessons from observational studies. *J Hypertens* 1998; **16**(Suppl):S3-7.

40. Pickering TG. Blood pressure measurement and detection of hypertension. *Lancet* 1994; **344**:31-5.

41. Mulrow PJ. Hypertension: a worldwide epidemic. In: Izzo JL, Black HR, Goodfriend TL, editors. *Hypertension primer: the essentials of high blood pressure.* 2nd ed. Baltimore (MD): Williams & Wilkins, 1999:271-3.

42. Joint National Committee on Prevention, Detection, Evaluation, and Treatment of High Blood Pressure. The sixth report of the Joint National Committee on Prevention, Detection, Evaluation, and Treatment of High Blood Pressure [published erratum appears in *Arch Intern Med* 1998; **158**:573]. *Arch Intern Med* 1997; **157**:2413-46.

43. Leitschuh M, Cupples LA, Kannel W, Gagnon D, Chobanian A. High-normal blood pressure progression to hypertension in the Framingham Heart Study. *Hypertension* 1991; **17**:22-7.

44. Kannel WB. Office assessment of coronary candidates and risk factor insights from the Framingham study. *J Hypertens* 1991; **9**(Suppl):S13-19.

45. Frost PH, Davis BR, Burlando AJ, *et al.* Coronary heart disease risk factors in men and women aged 60 years and older: findings from the Systolic Hypertension in the Elderly Program. *Circulation* 1996; **94**:26-34.

46. Pearson TA, LaCroix AZ, Mead LA, Liang KY. The prediction of midlife coronary heart disease and hypertension in young adults: the Johns Hopkins multiple risk equations. *Am J Prev Med* 1990; **6**:23-8.

47. Shinton R, Beevers G. Meta-analysis of relation between cigarette smoking and stroke. *BMJ* 1989; **298**:789-94.

48. Rich-Edwards JW, Manson JE, Hennekens CH, Buring JE. Medical progress: the primary prevention of coronary heart disease in women. *N Engl J Med* 1995; **332**:1758-66.

49. Kannel WB. Hypertension. Relationship with other risk factors. *Drugs* 1986; **31**:1-11.

50. Prescott E, Hippe M, Schnohr P, Hein HO, Vestbo J. Smoking and risk of myocardial infarction in women and men: longitudinal population study. *BMJ* 1998; **316**:1043-7.

51. Winkleby MA, Kraemer HC, Ahn DK, Varady AN. Ethnic and socioeconomic differences in cardiovascular disease risk factors: findings for women from the Third National Health and Nutrition Examination Survey, 1988-1994. *JAMA* 1998; **280**:356-62.

52. Keil JE, Sutherland SE, Knapp RG, Lackland DT, Gazes PC, Tyroler HA. Mortality rates and risk factors for coronary disease in black as compared with white men and women. *N Engl J Med* 1993; **329**:73-8.

53. Wei M, Mitchell BD, Haffner SM, Stern MP. Effects of cigarette smoking, diabetes, high cholesterol, and hypertension on all-cause mortality and cardiovascular disease mortality in Mexican Americans. The San Antonio Heart Study. *Am J Epidemiol* 1996; **144**:1058-65.

54. Roncaglioni MC, Santoro L, D'Avanzo B, *et al.* Role of family history in patients with myocardial infarction. An Italian case-control study. GISSI-EFRIM Investigators. *Circulation* 1992; **85**:2065-72.

55. Wilson PW, D'Agostino RB, Levy D, Belanger AM, Silbershatz H, Kannel WB. Prediction of coronary heart disease using risk factor categories. *Circulation* 1998; **97**:1837-47.

56. Neaton JD, Wentworth D. Serum cholesterol, blood pressure, cigarette smoking, and death from coronary heart disease. Overall findings and differences by age for 316,099 white men. Multiple Risk Factor Intervention Trial Research Group. *Arch Intern Med* 1992; **152**:56-64.

57. Wilson PW, Anderson KM, Castelli WP. Twelve-year incidence of coronary heart disease in middle-aged adults during the era of hypertensive therapy: the Framingham offspring study [published erratum appears in *Am J Med* 1991;**90**:537]. *Am J Med* 1991; **90**:11-16.

58. Hokanson JE, Austin MA. Plasma triglyceride level is a risk factor for cardiovascular disease independent of high-density lipoprotein cholesterol level: a meta-analysis of population-based prospective studies. *J Cardiovasc Risk* 1996; **3**:213-19.

59. Bostom AG, Gagnon DR, Cupples LA, *et al.* A prospective investigation of elevated lipoprotein (a) detected by electrophoresis and cardiovascular disease in women. The Framingham Heart Study. *Circulation* 1994; **90**:1688-95.

60. Hermanson B, Omenn GS, Kronmal RA, Gersh BJ. Beneficial six-year outcome of smoking cessation in older men and women with coronary artery disease. Results from the CASS registry. *N Engl J Med* 1988; **319**:1365-9.

61. Dagenais GR, Robitaille NM, Lupien PJ, *et al.* First coronary heart disease event rates in relation to major risk factors: Quebec cardiovascular study. *Can J Cardiol* 1990; **6**:274-80.

62. Benfante R, Reed D. Is elevated serum cholesterol level a risk factor for coronary heart disease in the elderly? *JAMA* 1990; **263**:393-6.

63. Kleinman JC, Donahue RP, Harris MI, Finucane FF, Madans JH, Brock DB. Mortality among diabetics in a national sample. *Am J Epidemiol* 1988; **128**:389-401.

64. Berlin JA, Colditz GA. A meta-analysis of physical activity in the prevention of coronary heart disease. *Am J Epidemiol* 1990; **132**:612-28.

65. Sandvik L, Erikssen J, Thaulow E, Erikssen G, Mundal R, Rodahl K. Physical fitness as a predictor of mortality among healthy, middle-aged Norwegian men. *N Engl J Med* 1993; **328**:533-7.

66. Hubert HB, Feinleib M, McNamara PM, Castelli WP. Obesity as an independent risk factor for cardiovascular disease: a 26-year follow-up of participants in the Framingham Heart Study. *Circulation* 1983; **67**:968-77.

67. Thun MJ, Peto R, Lopez AD, *et al.* Alcohol consumption and mortality among middle-aged and elderly U.S. adults. *N Engl J Med* 1997; **337**:1705-14.

68. Dunn FG, McLenachan J, Isles CG, *et al.* Left ventricular hypertrophy and mortality in hypertension: an analysis of data from the Glasgow Blood Pressure Clinic. *J Hypertens* 1990; **8**:775-82.

69. Levy D, Salomon M, D'Agostino RB, Belanger AJ, Kannel WB. Prognostic implications of baseline electrocardiographic features and their serial changes in subjects with left ventricular hypertrophy. *Circulation* 1994; **90**:1786-93.

70. Culleton BF, Larson MG, Kannel WB, Levy D. Serum uric acid and risk for cardiovascular disease and death: the Framingham Heart Study. *Ann Intern Med* 1999; **131**:7-13.

71. Ward HJ. Uric acid as an independent risk factor in the treatment of hypertension [published erratum appears in *Lancet* 1998; **352**:912]. *Lancet* 1998; **352**:670-1.

72. Alderman MH, Ooi WL, Cohen H, Madhavan S, Sealey JE, Laragh JH. Plasma renin activity: a risk factor for myocardial infarction in hypertensive patients. *Am J Hypertens* 1997; **10**:1-8.

73. Ernst E, Resch KL. Fibrinogen as a cardiovascular risk factor: a meta-analysis and review of the literature. *Ann Intern Med* 1993; **118**:956-63.

74. Danesh J, Lewington S. Plasma homocysteine and coronary heart disease: systematic review of published epidemiological studies. *J Cardiovasc Risk* 1998; **5**:229-32.

75. Boushey CJ, Beresford SA, Omenn GS, Motulsky AG. A quantitative assessment of plasma homocysteine as a risk factor for vascular disease. Probable benefits of increasing folic acid intakes. *JAMA* 1995; **274**:1049-57.

76. Stokes J 3d, Kannel WB, Wolf PA, Cupples LA, D'Agostino RB. The relative importance of selected risk factors for various manifestations of cardiovascular disease among men and women from 35 to 64 years old: 30 years of follow-up in the Framingham Study. *Circulation* 1987; **75**:V65-73.

77. MacMahon SW, Cutler JA, Furberg CD, Payne GH. The effects of drug treatment for hypertension on morbidity and mortality from cardiovascular disease: a review of randomized controlled trials. *Prog Cardiovasc Dis* 1986; **29**:99-118.

78. Tsevat J, Weinstein MC, Williams LW, Tosteson AN, Goldman L. Expected gains in life expectancy from various coronary heart disease risk factor modifications [published erratum appears in *Circulation* 1991; **84**:2610]. *Circulation* 1991; **83**:1194-201.

79. Blacher J, Staessen JA, Girerd X, *et al.* Pulse pressure not mean pressure determines cardiovascular risk in older hypertensive patients. *Arch Intern Med* 2000; **160**:1085-9.

80. Oparil S, Weber MA, editors. *Hypertension: a companion to Brenner and Rector's the kidney.* Philadelphia: W.B. Saunders, 2000.

81. Rutan GH, Kuller LH, Neaton JD, Wentworth DN, McDonald RH, Smith WM. Mortality associated with diastolic hypertension and isolated systolic hypertension among men screened for the Multiple Risk Factor Intervention Trial. *Circulation* 1988; **77**:504-14.

82. Franklin SS, Gustin W 4th, Wong ND, *et al.* Hemodynamic patterns of age-related changes in blood pressure. The Framingham Heart Study. *Circulation* 1997; **96**:308-15.

83. Abernethy J, Borhani NO, Hawkins CM, *et al.* Systolic blood pressure as an independent predictor of mortality in the Hypertension Detection and Follow-up Program. *Am J Prev Med* 1986; **2**:123-32.

84. Law MR, Wald NJ, Thompson SG. By how much and how quickly does reduction in serum cholesterol concentration lower risk of ischaemic heart disease? *BMJ* 1994; **308**:367-72.

85. LaRosa JC, He J, Vupputuri S. Effect of statins on risk of coronary disease: a meta-analysis of randomized controlled trials. *JAMA* 1999; **282**:2340-6.

86. Pignone M, Phillips C, Mulrow C. Use of lipid lowering drugs for primary prevention of coronary heart disease: meta-analysis of randomised trials. *BMJ* 2000; **321**:983-6.

87. Avins AL, Neuhaus JM. Do triglycerides provide meaningful information about heart disease risk? *Arch Intern Med* 2000; **160**:1937-44.

88. Goldbourt U, Brunner D, Behar S, Reicher-Reiss H. Baseline characteristics of patients participating in the Bezafibrate Infarction Prevention (BIP) Study. *Eur Heart J* 1998; **19**:H42-7.

89. De Faire U, Ericsson CG, Grip L, Nilsson J, Svane B, Hamsten A. Secondary preventive potential of lipid-lowering drugs. The Bezafibrate Coronary Atherosclerosis Intervention Trial (BECAIT). *Eur Heart J* 1996; **17** (Suppl F):37-42.

90. Rubins HB, Robins SJ, Collins D, *et al.* Gemfibrozil for the secondary prevention of coronary heart disease in men with low levels of high-density lipoprotein cholesterol. Veterans Affairs High-Density Lipoprotein Cholesterol Intervention Trial Study Group. *N Engl J Med* 1999; **341**:410-18.

91. Scanu AM, Fless GM. Lipoprotein (a). Heterogeneity and biological relevance. *J Clin Invest* 1990; **85**:1709-15.

92. Rader DJ, Hoeg JM, Brewer HB Jr. Quantitation of plasma apolipoproteins in the primary and secondary prevention of coronary artery disease. *Ann Intern Med* 1994; **120**:1012-25.

93. Harjai KJ. Potential new cardiovascular risk factors: left ventricular hypertrophy, homocysteine, lipoprotein(a), triglycerides, oxidative stress, and fibrinogen. *Ann Intern Med* 1999; **131**:376-86.

94. Ridker PM, Hennekens CH, Stampfer MJ. A prospective study of lipoprotein(a) and the risk of myocardial infarction. *JAMA* 1993; **270**:2195-9.

95. Ridker PM, Stampfer MJ, Hennekens CH. Plasma concentration of lipoprotein(a) and the risk of future stroke. *JAMA* 1995; **273**:1269-73.

96. Sechi LA, Kronenberg F, De Carli S, *et al*. Association of serum lipoprotein(a) levels and apolipoprotein(a) size polymorphism with target-organ damage in arterial hypertension. *JAMA* 1997; **277**:1689-95.

97. Kannel WB, Higgins M. Smoking and hypertension as predictors of cardiovascular risk in population studies. *J Hypertens* 1990; **8**(Suppl):S3-8.

98. Iribarren C, Tekawa IS, Sidney S, Friedman GD. Effect of cigar smoking on the risk of cardiovascular disease, chronic obstructive pulmonary disease, and cancer in men. *N Engl J Med* 1999; **340**:1773-80.

99. United States Public Health Service. Office of the Surgeon General. *The health benefits of smoking cessation: a report of the Surgeon General*. Rockville (MD): U.S. Department of Health and Human Services, Center for Chronic Disease Prevention and Health Promotion, Office on Smoking and Health, 1990. DHHS publication; no. (CDC) 90-8416.

100. Royal College of Physicians of London. *Smoking and health now: a new report and summary on smoking and its effects on health*. London, England: Pittman Medical and Scientific Pub. Co, 1971.

101. Wilson PW. Established risk factors and coronary artery disease: the Framingham Study. *Am J Hypertens* 1994; **7**:7S-12S.

102. Kannel WB, Neaton JD, Wentworth D, *et al*. Overall and coronary heart disease mortality rates in relation to major risk factors in 325,348 men screened for the MRFIT. Multiple Risk Factor Intervention Trial. *Am Heart J* 1986; **112**:825-36.

103. The Diabetes Control and Complications Trial Research Group. The effect of intensive treatment of diabetes on the development and progression of long-term complications in insulin-dependent diabetes mellitus. *N Engl J Med* 1993; **329**:977-86.

104. UK Prospective Diabetes Study (UKPDS) Group. Intensive blood-glucose control with sulphonylureas or insulin compared with conventional treatment and risk of complications in patients with type 2 diabetes (UKPDS 33) [published erratum appears in *Lancet* 1999; **354**:602]. *Lancet* 1998; **352**:837-53.

105. Dannenberg AL, Keller JB, Wilson PW, Castelli WP. Leisure time physical activity in the Framingham Offspring Study. Description, seasonal variation, and risk factor correlates. *Am J Epidemiol* 1989; **129**:76-88.

106. Pekkanen J, Marti B, Nissinen A, Tuomilehto J, Punsar S, Karvonen MJ. Reduction of premature mortality by high physical activity: a 20-year follow-up of middle-aged Finnish men. *Lancet* 1987; **i**:1473-7.

107. Meade TW, Chakrabarti R, Haines AP, North WR, Stirling Y. Characteristics affecting fibrinolytic activity and plasma fibrinogen concentrations. *BMJ* 1979; **i**:153-6.

108. Alexander JK. Obesity and cardiac performance. *Am J Cardiol* 1964; **14**:860-5.

109. Tuomilehto J. Body mass index and prognosis in elderly hypertensive patients: a report from the European Working Party on High Blood Pressure in the Elderly. *Am J Med* 1991; **90**:34S-41S.

110. Stamler R, Ford CE, Stamler J. Why do lean hypertensives have higher mortality rates than other hypertensives? Findings of the Hypertension Detection and Follow-up Program. *Hypertension* 1991; **17**:553-64.

111. Hartz AJ, Rupley DC, Rimm AA. The association of girth measurements with disease in 32856 women. *Am J Epidemiol* 1984; **119**:71-80.

112. Peiris AN, Sothmann MS, Hoffmann RG, *et al*. Adiposity, fat distribution, and cardiovascular risk. *Ann Intern Med* 1989; **110**:867-72.

113. Gillum RF. The association of body fat distribution with hypertension, hypertensive heart disease, coronary heart disease, diabetes and cardiovascular risk factors in men and women aged 18-79 years. *J Chronic Dis* 1987; **40**:421-8.

114. Welin L, Svardsudd K, Wilhelmsen L, Larsson B, Tibblin G. Analysis of risk factors for stroke in a cohort of men born in 1913. *N Engl J Med* 1987; **317**:521-6.

115. Lapidus L, Bengtsson C, Larsson B, Pennert K, Rybo E, Sjostrom L. Distribution of adipose tissue and risk of cardiovascular disease and death: a 12 year follow up of participants in the population study of women in Gothenburg, Sweden. *BMJ* 1984; **289**:1257-61.

116. Walker SP, Rimm EB, Ascherio A, Kawachi I, Stampfer MJ, Willett WC. Body size and fat distribution as predictors of stroke among US men. *Am J Epidemiol* 1996; **144**:1143-50.

117. Folsom AR, Prineas RJ, Kaye SA, Soler JT. Body fat distribution and self-reported prevalence of hypertension, heart attack, and other heart disease in older women. *Int J Epidemiol* 1989; **18**:361-7.

118. Hartz A, Grubb B, Wild R, *et al.* The association of waist hip ratio and angiographically determined coronary artery disease. *Int J Obes* 1990; **14**:657-65.

119. Folsom AR, Prineas RJ, Kaye SA, Munger RG. Incidence of hypertension and stroke in relation to body fat distribution and other risk factors in older women. *Stroke* 1990; **21**:701-6.

120. National Institutes of Health. *Clinical guidelines on the identification, evaluation, and treatment of overweight and obesity in adults : the evidence report.* Bethesda (MD): National Heart, Lung, and Blood Institute in cooperation with the National Institute of Diabetes and Digestive and Kidney Disease, 1998. NIH publication: no. 98-4083.

121. Boffetta P, Garfinkel L. Alcohol drinking and mortality among men enrolled in an American Cancer Society prospective study. *Epidemiology* 1990; **1**:342-8.

122. Doll R, Peto R, Hall E, Wheatley K, Gray R. Mortality in relation to consumption of alcohol: 13 years' observations on male British doctors. *BMJ* 1994; **309**:911-18.

123. Marmot MG, Rose G, Shipley MJ, Thomas BJ. Alcohol and mortality: a U-shaped curve. *Lancet* 1981; **i**:580-3.

124. Suh I, Shaten BJ, Cutler JA, Kuller LH. Alcohol use and mortality from coronary heart disease: the role of high-density lipoprotein cholesterol. The Multiple Risk Factor Intervention Trial Research Group. *Ann Intern Med* 1992; **116**:881-7.

125. Boffetta P, Garfinkel L. Alcohol drinking and mortality among men enrolled in an American Cancer Society prospective study. *Epidemiology* 1990; **1**:342-8.

126. Kannel WB. Left ventricular hypertrophy as a risk factor: the Framingham experience. *J Hypertens* 1991; **9**(Suppl):S3-9.

127. Devereux RB, Roman MJ. Left ventricular hypertrophy in hypertension: stimuli, patterns, and consequences. *Hypertens Res* 1999; **22**:1-9.

128. Koren MJ, Devereux RB, Casale PN, Savage DD, Laragh JH. Relation of left ventricular mass and geometry to morbidity and mortality in uncomplicated essential hypertension. *Ann Intern Med* 1991; **114**:345-52.

129. Casale PN, Devereux RB, Milner M, *et al.* Value of echocardiographic measurement of left ventricular mass in predicting cardiovascular morbid events in hypertensive men. *Ann Intern Med* 1986; **105**:173-8.

130. Devereux RB, de Simone G, Ganau A, Roman MJ. Left ventricular hypertrophy and geometric remodeling in hypertension: stimuli, functional consequences and prognostic implications. *J Hypertens* 1994; **12**(Suppl):S117-27.

131. Schmieder RE, Martus P, Klingbeil A. Reversal of left ventricular hypertrophy in essential hypertension. A meta-analysis of randomized double-blind studies. *JAMA* 1996; **275**:1507-13.

132. Verdecchia P, Schillaci G, Borgioni C, *et al.* Prognostic significance of serial changes in left ventricular mass in essential hypertension. *Circulation* 1998; **97**:48-54.

133. Ljungman S. Microalbuminuria in essential hypertension. *Am J Hypertens* 1990; **3**:956-60.

134. Mimran A. Microalbuminuria in essential hypertension. *Clin Exp Hypertens* 1997; **19**:753-67.

135. Luft FC, Agrawal B. Microalbuminuria as a predictive factor for cardiovascular events. *J Cardiovasc Pharmacol* 1999; **33**(Suppl) **1**:S11-5.

136. Pontremoli R, Viazzi F, Sofia A, *et al*. Microalbuminuria: a marker of cardiovascular risk and organ damage in essential hypertension. *Kidney Int* 1997; **63**(Suppl):S163-5.

137. Pontremoli R, Cheli V, Sofia A, *et al*. Prevalence of micro- and macroalbuminuria and their relationship with other cardiovascular risk factors in essential hypertension. *Nephrol Dial Transplant* 1995; **10**:6-9.

138. Bigazzi R, Bianchi S, Baldari D, Campese VM. Microalbuminuria predicts cardiovascular events and renal insufficiency in patients with essential hypertension. *J Hypertens* 1998; **16**:1325-33.

139. Ljungman S, Wikstrand J, Hartford M, Berglund G. Urinary albumin excretion — a predictor of risk of cardiovascular disease. A prospective 10-year follow-up of middle-aged nondiabetic normal and hypertensive men. *Am J Hypertens* 1996; **9**:770-8.

140. Agewall S, Persson B, Samuelsson O, Ljungman S, Herlitz H, Fagerberg B. Microalbuminuria in treated hypertensive men at high risk of coronary disease. The Risk Factor Intervention Study Group. *J Hypertens* 1993; **11**:461-9.

141. Bianchi S, Bigazzi R, Campese VM. Microalbuminuria in essential hypertension. *J Nephrol* 1997; **10**:216-19.

142. Janssen WM, De Jong PE, De Zeeuw D. Hypertension and renal disease: role of microalbuminuria. *J Hypertens* 1996; **14**(Suppl):S173-7.

143. Bigazzi R, Bianchi S, Baldari D, Sgherri G, Baldari G, Campese VM. Microalbuminuria in salt-sensitive patients. A marker for renal and cardiovascular risk factors. *Hypertension* 1994; **23**:195-9.

144. Jensen JS, Feldt-Rasmussen B, Borch-Johnsen K, Clausen P, Appleyard M, Jensen G. Microalbuminuria and its relation to cardiovascular disease and risk factors. A population-based study of 1254 hypertensive individuals. *J Hum Hypertens* 1997; **11**:727-32.

145. Agewall S, Wikstrand J, Ljungman S, Fagerberg B. Usefulness of microalbuminuria in predicting cardiovascular mortality in treated hypertensive men with and without diabetes mellitus. Risk Factor Intervention Study Group. *Am J Cardiol* 1997; **80**:164-9.

146. Alderman MH, Cohen H, Madhavan S, Kivlighn S. Serum uric acid and cardiovascular events in successfully treated hypertensive patients. *Hypertension* 1999; **34**:144-50.

147. Beevers DG, Lip GY. Is uric acid really an independent cardiovascular risk factor? *Lancet* 1998; **352**:1556.

148. Staessen J. The determinants and prognostic significance of serum uric acid in elderly patients of the European Working Party on High Blood Pressure in the Elderly trial. *Am J Med* 1991; **90**:50S-4S.

149. Lee AJ, Lowe GD, Woodward M, Tunstall-Pedoe H. Fibrinogen in relation to personal history of prevalent hypertension, diabetes, stroke, intermittent claudication, coronary heart disease, and family history: the Scottish Heart Health Study. *Br Heart J* 1993; **69**:338-42.

150. Behar S. Lowering fibrinogen levels: clinical update. BIP Study Group. Bezafibrate Infarction Prevention. *Blood Coagul Fibrinolysis* 1999; **10**:S41-3.

151. Graham I. Homocysteine in health and disease. *Ann Intern Med* 1999; **131**:387-8.

152. Eikelboom JW, Lonn E, Genest J Jr, Hankey G, Yusuf S. Homocyst(e)ine and cardiovascular disease: a critical review of the epidemiologic evidence. *Ann Intern Med* 1999; **131**:363-75.

153. Koenig W. Heart disease and the inflammatory response. Although it's an integral part of the atherosclerotic process we still don't know why. *BMJ* 2000; **321**:187-8.

154. Fagerberg B, Gnarpe J, Gnarpe H, Agewall S, Wikstrand J. Chlamydia pneumoniae but not cytomegalovirus antibodies are associated with future risk of stroke and cardiovascular disease: a prospective study in middle-aged to elderly men with treated hypertension. *Stroke* 1999; **30**:299-305.

155. Wald NJ, Law MR, Morris JK, Zhou X, Wong Y, Ward ME. Chlamydia pneumoniae infection and mortality from ischaemic heart disease: large prospective study. *BMJ* 2000; **321**:204-7.

156. Danesh J, Whincup P, Walker M, *et al.* Chlamydia pneumoniae IgG titres and coronary heart disease: prospective study and meta-analysis. *BMJ* 2000; **321**:208-13.

157. Danesh J, Whincup P, Walker M, *et al.* Low grade inflammation and coronary heart disease: prospective study and updated meta-analyses. *BMJ* 2000; **321**:199-204.

158. Materson BJ. Will angiotensin converting enzyme genotype, receptor mutation identification, and other miracles of molecular biology permit reduction of NNT? *Am J Hypertens* 1998; **11**:138S-42S.

159. McAlister FA, Laupacis A. Towards a better yardstick: the choice of treatment thresholds in hypertension. *Can J Cardiol* 1998; **14**:47-51.

160. Eriksson H, Welin L, Wilhelmsen L, *et al.* Metabolic disturbances in hypertension: results from the population study 'men born in 1913'. *J Intern Med* 1992; **232**:389-95.

161. Kaplan NM. Multiple risk factors for coronary heart disease in patients with hypertension. *J Hypertens* 1995; **13**(Suppl):S1-5.

162. Kannel WB. Cardioprotection and antihypertensive therapy: the key importance of addressing the associated coronary risk factors (the Framingham experience). *Am J Cardiol* 1996; **77**:6B-11B.

163. Rantala AO, Kauma H, Lilja M, Savolainen MJ, Reunanen A, Kesaniemi YA. Prevalence of the metabolic syndrome in drug-treated hypertensive patients and control subjects. *J Intern Med* 1999; **245**:163-74.

164. Alderman MH. Quantifying cardiovascular risk in hypertension. *Cardiol Clin* 1995; **13**:519-27.

165. Jackson R, Barham P, Bills J, *et al.* Management of raised blood pressure in New Zealand: a discussion document. *BMJ* 1993; **307**:107-10.

166. Wolf PA, D'Agostino RB, Belanger AJ, Kannel WB. Probability of stroke: a risk profile from the Framingham Study. *Stroke* 1991; **22**:312-18.

167. Kannel WB, D'Agostino RB, Silbershatz H, Belanger AJ, Wilson PW, Levy D. Profile for estimating risk of heart failure. *Arch Intern Med* 1999; **159**:1197-204.

168. Truett J, Cornfield J, Kannel W. A multivariate analysis of the risk of coronary heart disease in Framingham. *J Chronic Dis* 1967; **20**:511-24.

169. Haq IU, Ramsay LE, Yeo WW, Jackson PR, Wallis EJ. Is the Framingham risk function valid for northern European populations? A comparison of methods for estimating absolute coronary risk in high risk men. *Heart* 1999; **81**:40-6.

170. The West of Scotland Coronary Prevention Study Group. Baseline risk factors and their association with outcome in the West of Scotland Coronary Prevention Study. *Am J Cardiol* 1997; **79**:756-62.

171. Schulte H, Assmann G. CHD risk equations, obtained from the Framingham heart study, applied to the PROCAM study. *Cardiovas Risk Factors* 1991; **1**:126-33.

172. SBU: Swedish Council on Technology Assessment in Health Care. Moderately elevated blood pressure. A report from SBU, the Swedish Council on Technology Assessment in Health Care. *J Intern Med* 1995; **238**(Suppl):1-225.

173. Durrington PN, Prais H, Bhatnagar D, *et al.* Indications for cholesterol-lowering medication: comparison of risk-assessment methods [published erratum appears in *Lancet* 1999; **354**:166]. *Lancet* 1999; **353**:278-81.

174. Haq IU, Jackson PR, Yeo WW, Ramsay LE. Sheffield risk and treatment table for cholesterol lowering for primary prevention of coronary heart disease. *Lancet* 1995; **346**:1467-71.

175. Pyorala K, De Backer G, Graham I, Poole-Wilson P, Wood D. Prevention of coronary heart disease in clinical practice. Recommendations of the Task Force of the European Society of Cardiology, European Atherosclerosis Society and European Society of Hypertension. *Eur Heart J* 1994; **15**:1300-31.

176. Laurier D, Nguyen PC, Cazelles B, Segond P. Estimation of CHD risk in a French working population using a modified Framingham model. The PCV-METRA Group. *J Clin Epidemiol* 1994; **47**:1353-64.

177. Gordon T, Garcia-Palmieri MR, Kagan A, Kannel WB, Schiffman J. Differences in coronary heart disease in Framingham, Honolulu and Puerto Rico. *J Chronic Dis* 1974; **27**:329-44.

178. Keys A, Menotti A, Aravanis C, *et al.* The seven countries study: 2289 deaths in 15 years. *Prev Med* 1984; **13**:141-54.

179. Grover SA, Paquet S, Levinton C, Coupal L, Zowall H. Estimating the benefits of modifying risk factors of cardiovascular disease: a comparison of primary vs secondary prevention [published erratum appears in *Arch Intern Med* 1998;**158**:1228]. *Arch Intern Med* 1998; **158**:655-62.

180. Tunstall-Pedoe H. The Dundee coronary risk-disk for management of change in risk factors. *BMJ* 1991; **303**:744-7.

181. Assman G. *Lipid metabolism disorders and coronary heart disease: primary prevention, diagnosis, and therapy guidelines for general practice.* 2nd ed. München, Germany: MMV Medizin Verlag, 1993.

182. Shaper AG, Pocock SJ, Phillips AN, Walker M. Identifying men at high risk of heart attacks: strategy for use in general practice. *BMJ* 1986; **293**:474-9.

183. McAlister FA, Laupacis A, Teo KK, Hamilton PG, Montague TJ. A survey of clinician attitudes and management practices in hypertension. *J Hum Hypertens* 1997; **11**:413-19.

184. McAlister FA, Teo KK, Lewanczuk RZ, Wells G, Montague TJ. Contemporary practice patterns in the management of newly diagnosed hypertension. *CMAJ* 1997; **157**:23-30.

185. Laupacis A, Sackett DL, Roberts RS. An assessment of clinically useful measures of the consequences of treatment. *N Engl J Med* 1988; **318**:1728-33.

186. Laupacis A, Sackett DL, Roberts RS. Therapeutic priorities of Canadian internists. *CMAJ* 1990; **142**:329-33.

187. Linjer E, Hansson L. Underestimation of the true benefits of antihypertensive treatment: an assessment of some important sources of error. *J Hypertens* 1997; **15**:221-5.

188. McAlister FA, O'Connor AM, Wells G, Grover SA, Laupacis A. When should hypertension be treated? The different perspectives of Canadian family physicians and patients. *CMAJ* 2000;**163**:403-8.

189. Steel N. Thresholds for taking antihypertensive drugs in different professional and lay groups: questionnaire survey. *BMJ* 2000; **320**:1446-7.

190. McAlister FA, Straus SE, Guyatt GH, Haynes RB. Users' guides to the medical literature: XX. Integrating research evidence with the care of the individual patient. Evidence-based Medicine Working Group. *JAMA* 2000; **283**:2829-36.

191. Ramsay LE, Haq IU, Yeo WW, Jackson PR. Interpretation of prospective trials in hypertension: do treatment guidelines accurately reflect current evidence? *J Hypertens* 1996; **14**(Suppl):S187-94.

192. Jaeschke R, Singer J, Guyatt GH. Measurement of health status. Ascertaining the minimal clinically important difference. *Control Clin Trials* 1989; **10**:407-15.

193. O'Connor AM, Rostom A, Fiset V, *et al.* Decision aids for patients facing health treatment or screening decisions: systematic review. *BMJ* 1999; **319**:731-4.

194. Deber RB, Kraetschmer N, Irvine J. What role do patients wish to play in treatment decision making? *Arch Intern Med* 1996; **156**:1414-20.

Acknowledgements

The authors thank Ms Shirley Osborne for her assistance in obtaining and collating the references.

Appendix 1: Assessing coronary heart disease risk for women

These score sheets are based on women aged 30 to 74 years in the Framingham cohort. Work through Steps 1 through 6 for individual patients. Add points derived from each Step 1 through 6 to reach a total score for the individual patient (Step 7). Step 8 shows how the patient's score relates to her 10-year risk for coronary heart disease. Step 9 shows the comparative average risks for other women in her age group.

Step 1		
Age		
Years	LDL points	Cholesterol points
30 to 34	–9	[–9]
35 to 39	–4	[–4]
40 to 44	0	[0]
45 to 49	3	[3]
50 to 54	6	[6]
55 to 59	7	[7]
60 to 64	8	[8]
65 to 69	8	[8]
70 to 74	9	[9]

Step 2		
LDL-C		
(mg/dL)	(mmol/L)	LDL points
≤ 99	≤ 2.59	–3
100 to 129	2.60 to 3.36	0
130 to 159	3.37 to 4.14	0
160 to 189	4.15 to 4.91	1
≥ 190	≥ 4.92	2
Cholesterol		
(mg/dL)	(mmol/L)	Cholesterol points
< 160	< 4.14	[–3]
160 to 199	4.15 to 5.17	[0]
200 to 239	5.18 to 6.21	[1]
240 to 279	6.22 to 7.24	[2]
≥ 280	≥ 7.25	[3]

Step 3

HDL-C

(md/dL)	(mmol/L)	LDL points	Cholesterol points
< 35	< 0.90	2	[2]
35 to 44	0.91 to 1.16	1	[1]
45 to 49	1.17 to 1.29	0	[0]
50 to 59	1.30 to 1.55	0	[0]
≥ 60	≥ 1.56	−1	[−2]

Step 4

Blood pressure

Systolic (mm Hg)	Diastolic (mm Hg)				
	< 80	80 to 84	85 to 89	90 to 99	≥ 100
< 120	0 [0] points				
120 to 129		0 [0] points			
130 to 139			1 [1] points		
140 to 159				2 [2] points	
> 160					3 [3] points

When systolic and diastolic pressures provide different estimates for point scores, use the higher number.

Step 5

Diabetes

	LDL points	Cholesterol points
No	0	[0]
Yes	2	[2]

Step 6

Smoker

	LDL points	Cholesterol points
No	0	[0]
Yes	2	[2]

Step 7

Adding up the points

Age	
LDL-C or cholesterol	
HDL-C	
Blood pressure	
Diabetes	
Smoker	
Point total	

Step 8

Coronary heart disease risk

LDL points total	10-Year CHD risk	Cholesterol points total	10-Year CHD risk
≤ −3	1%		
−2	2%		
−1	2%	[<−1]	[2%]
0	3%	[0]	[3%]
1	4%	[1]	[3%]
2	4%	[2]	[4%]
3	5%	[3]	[5%]
4	7%	[4]	[7%]
5	9%	[5]	[8%]
6	11%	[6]	[10%]
7	14%	[7]	[13%]
8	18%	[8]	[16%]
9	22%	[9]	[20%]
10	27%	[10]	[25%]
11	33%	[11]	[31%]
12	40%	[12]	[37%]
13	47%	[13]	[45%]
≥14	≥56%	[≥14]	[≥53%]

Step 9

Comparative risk

Age (years)	Average 10-year CHD risk	Average 10-year hard[a] CHD risk	Low[b] 10-year CHD risk
30 to 34	< 3%	< 1%	< 1%
35 to 39	< 1%	< 1%	1%
40 to 44	2%	1%	2%
45 to 49	5%	2%	3%
50 to 54	8%	3%	5%
55 to 59	12%	7%	7%
60 to 64	12%	8%	8%
65 to 69	13%	8%	8%
70 to 74	14%	11%	8%

[a]Hard events exclude angina pectoris.

[b]Low risk was calculated for a person the same age, optimal blood pressure, LDL-C 100 to 129 mg/dL or cholesterol 160 to 199 mg/dL, HDL-C 45 mg/dL for men, nonsmoker, and no diabetes.

Reproduced with permission from Wilson PW, D'Agostino RB, Levy D, Belangor AM. Prediction of coronary heart disease using risk factor categories. Circulation 1998;**97**:1837-47.

Appendix 2: Assessing coronary heart disease risk for men

These score sheets are based on men aged 30 to 74 years in the Framingham cohort. Work through Steps 1 through 6 for individual patients. Add points derived from each Step 1 through 6 to reach a total score for the individual patient (Step 7). Step 8 shows how the patient's score relates to his 10-year risk for coronary heart disease. Step 9 shows the comparative average risks for other men in his age group.

Step 1		
Age		
Years	**LDL points**	**Cholesterol points**
30 to 34	−1	[−1]
35 to 39	0	[0]
40 to 44	1	[1]
45 to 49	2	[2]
50 to 54	3	[3]
55 to 59	4	[4]
60 to 64	5	[5]
65 to 69	6	[6]
70 to 74	7	[7]

Step 2		
LDL-C		
(mg/dL)	**(mmol/L)**	**LDL points**
< 100	< 2.60	−3
100 to 129	2.60 to 3.36	0
130 to 159	3.37 to 4.14	0
160 to 189	4.15 to 4.91	1
≥ 190	≥ 4.92	2
Cholesterol		
(mg/dL)	**(mmol/L)**	**Cholesterol points**
< 160	< 4.14	[−3]
160 to 199	4.15 to 5.17	[0]
200 to 239	5.18 to 6.21	[1]
240 to 279	6.22 to 7.24	[2]
≥ 280	≥ 7.25	[3]

Step 3

HDL-C

(md/dL)	(mmol/L)	LDL points	Cholesterol points
< 35	< 0.90	2	[2]
35 to 44	0.91 to 1.16	1	[1]
45 to 49	1.17 to 1.29	0	[0]
50 to 59	1.30 to 1.55	0	[0]
≥ 60	≥ 1.56	–1	[–2]

Step 4

Blood pressure

Systolic (mm Hg)	Diastolic (mm Hg)				
	< 80	80 to 84	85 to 89	90 to 99	≥ 100
< 120	0 [0] points				
120 to 129		0 [0] points			
130 to 139			1 [1] points		
140 to 159				2 [2] points	
> 160					3 [3] points

When systolic and diastolic pressures provide different estimates for point scores, use the higher number.

Step 5

Diabetes

	LDL points	Cholesterol points
No	0	[0]
Yes	2	[2]

Step 6

Smoker

	LDL points	Cholesterol points
No	0	[0]
Yes	2	[2]

Step 7	
Adding up the points	
Age	
LDL-C or cholesterol	
HDL-C	
Blood pressure	
Diabetes	
Smoker	
Point total	

Step 8			
Coronary heart disease risk			
LDL points total	**10-Year CHD risk**	**Cholesterol points total**	**10-Year CHD risk**
≤ –3	1%		
–2	2%		
–1	2%	[<–1]	[2%]
0	3%	[0]	[3%]
1	4%	[1]	[3%]
2	4%	[2]	[4%]
3	5%	[3]	[5%]
4	7%	[4]	[7%]
5	9%	[5]	[8%]
6	11%	[6]	[10%]
7	14%	[7]	[13%]
8	18%	[8]	[16%]
9	22%	[9]	[20%]
10	27%	[10]	[25%]
11	33%	[11]	[31%]
12	40%	[12]	[37%]
13	47%	[13]	[45%]
≥14	≥56%	[≥14]	[≥53%]

Step 9

Comparative risk

Age (years)	Average 10-year CHD risk	Average 10-year hard[a] CHD risk	Low[b] 10-year CHD risk
30 to 34	3%	1%	2%
35 to 39	5%	4%	3%
40 to 44	7%	4%	4%
45 to 49	11%	8%	4%
50 to 54	14%	10%	6%
55 to 59	15%	13%	7%
60 to 64	21%	20%	9%
65 to 69	25%	22%	11%
70 to 74	30%	25%	14%

[a]Hard events exclude angina pectoris.

[b]Low risk was calculated for a person the same age, optimal blood pressure, LDL-C 100 to 129 mg/dL or cholesterol 160 to 199 mg/dL, HDL-C 45 mg/dL for men, nonsmoker, and no diabetes.

Reproduced with permission from Wilson PW, D'Agostino RB, Levy D, Belangor AM. Prediction of coronary heart disease using risk factor categories. Circulation 1998;**97**:1837-47.

CHAPTER 4

What are the elements of good treatment for hypertension?

Cynthia D Mulrow
Michael Pignone

What are the goals of treating patients with hypertension?

What are the therapeutic options for managing patients with high blood pressure?

What are the benefits and harms of antihypertensive drug therapy for people with hypertension?

What are the benefits and harms of treating dyslipidemia in people with hypertension?

What are the benefits and harms of smoking cessation in people with hypertension?

What are the benefits and harms of routine physical activity in people with hypertension?

What are the benefits and harms of particular dietary interventions in people with hypertension?

What are the benefits and harms of weight loss for hypertensive overweight patients?

What are the benefits and harms of antiplatelet treatment in people with hypertension?

What are the benefits and harms of modest alcohol consumption in people with hypertension?

What are the benefits and harms of anticoagulant treatment in people with hypertension?

What are the benefits and harms of various antioxidants and vitamins for people with hypertension?

What are the benefits and harms of garlic, potassium, calcium, and magnesium supplementation in people with hypertension?

Summary bottom lines

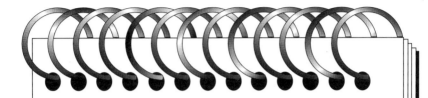

Patient Notes

Mr Willie Maykit, age 68, retired

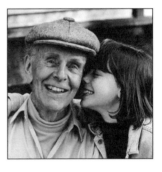

- Hypertension and diabetes; both well controlled
- Medications: ACE inhibitor, metformin and aspirin
- Supplements: multivitamin with ß-carotene, calcium and magnesium tablets, and fish oil

Reason for visit

- Wants reassurance that he is doing everything he can to stay healthy

Clinical findings

- BP 130/78 mm Hg, HgA1c 6.8

Clinical question

What therapies are likely to decrease rather than increase morbid and mortal clinical events in patients with hypertension?

What are the goals of treating patients with hypertension?

The following are our goals in treatment decisions:

- Decrease the attendant cardiovascular risk associated with hypertension
- Decrease the attendant risk of any coexisting cardiovascular risk factors
- Improve quality of life and encourage healthy lifestyles
- Choose therapeutic agents that are likely to do more good than harm given each individual's mix of social circumstances, preferences, coexisting medical conditions, and concomitant risk factors
- Minimize adverse effects and inconveniences of prescribed therapies.

 ## What are the therapeutic options for managing patients with high blood pressure?

Multiple options are available to help patients manage their hypertension and attendant cardiovascular risk. Tables 4.1 and 4.2 display a potpourri of these options that could be considered singly or in combination, depending upon the patient's mix of comorbid risk factors. Table 4.1 specifies options for patients without known cardiovascular disease; Table 4.2 specifies options for patients with known cardiovascular disease. We classify options in the following way:

- **Effective.** Multiple large randomized controlled trials or multiple large cohort studies consistently show options decrease rather than increase the incidence of major morbid and mortal events.
- **Possibly effective.** Some, but less, evidence from large trials and cohort studies that suggest improvements in clinical outcomes or evidence of close trade-offs between potential benefits and harms.
- **Unclearly effective.** No effects on clinically important outcomes are demonstrated or data are conflicting.
- **Probably ineffective.** Multiple trials or cohort studies consistently show the options do not decrease the incidence of major morbid and mortal events.
- **Possibly harmful.** Trials, cohort or case-control studies consistently suggest options lead to increases rather than decreases in major morbid and mortal events.

Table 4.1. Therapeutic options for people with hypertension and no known cardiovascular disease.

Effective	Possibly effective	Unclear	Probably ineffective	Possibly harmful
Antihypertensive drug therapies	Weight loss	Anticoagulant treatment	Vitamin E	Alpha-agonists
Lipid therapy	Diabetes management	Diet modification		Short-acting calcium channel blockers
Smoking cessation	Modest alcohol consumption	Antioxidants, vitamin C, fish oil, flavanoids		ß-carotene supplements
Physical activity	Antiplatelet treatment	Garlic, potassium, calcium, magnesium		

Table 4.2. Therapeutic options for people with hypertension and known cardiovascular disease.

Effective	Possibly effective	Unclear	Probably ineffective	Possibly harmful
Antihypertensive drug therapies	Mediterranean diet	Antioxidants	Vitamin E	Alpha-agonists
Lipid therapy	Diabetes management	Vitamin C, flavanoids		Short-acting calcium channel blockers
Smoking cessation	Modest alcohol consumption	Garlic, potassium, calcium, magnesium		ß-carotene supplements
Physical activity	Fish oil			
Antiplatelet treatment				
Anticoagulant treatment				

What are the benefits and harms of antihypertensive drug therapy for people with hypertension?

Benefits of antihypertensive treatment

We found multiple, large randomized placebo-controlled trials that consistently showed antihypertensive drug treatment decreased the risk of fatal and nonfatal stroke, cardiac events, and death in men and women with systolic or diastolic hypertension.[1,2](Tx: IIa) We also found randomized trials that showed quality of life is not adversely affected and may be improved with antihypertensive drug treatment.[3,4](Tx: IIb)

We found that the systolic and diastolic blood pressure reductions achieved in the trials varied but averaged around 10 to 15/5 to 10 mm Hg.

We found greater absolute benefits of drug treatment were seen among people with higher baseline cardiovascular risk, such as older adults with some comorbid risk factors. For example, on average, every 1000 patient years of treatment in older adults prevented five strokes (95% CI 2 to 8), three coronary events (95% CI 1 to 4), and four cardiovascular deaths (95% CI 1 to 8). Drug treatment in middle-aged adults prevented one stroke (95% CI 0 to 2) for every 1000 patient years of treatment and did not significantly affect coronary events or mortality.[5]

Benefits of specific antihypertensive drugs as first-line agents

We are unclear regarding whether benefits of specific antihypertensive drug therapies are closely tied to their effects on blood pressure or whether they are due to other multiple, heterogeneous effects of specific agents. We find it difficult to assess effects of particular agents because most large trials have tested stepped-care approaches where second and third drugs are added if a prespecified target blood pressure is not met. Below, we summarize data regarding particular agents used as first-line agents.

Thiazide diuretics

We found many of the large hypertension trials have compared hydrochlorothiazide, chlorthalidone, or a combination thiazide and potassium-sparing agent (e.g., amiloride or triamterene) with placebo or no drug therapy. Both low-dose and high-dose thiazide regimens decreased rates of stroke and death; only low-dose regimens had demonstrated efficacy in reducing coronary artery disease.[6](Tx: IIa) Evidence of effectiveness appeared consistent across several different thiazides, which suggested benefits are a class effect.

Beta-blockers

We found reviews of several randomized trials that compared beta-blockers as first-line antihypertensive agents with placebo.[7-10](Tx: LIb, L2b) We found these data were complicated. In some trials, as many as 70% of participants also received diuretics; in some trials, there were large numbers of participants who crossed over to other regimens. Regardless, data suggest, but do not prove, beta-blockers may reduce strokes but not coronary artery disease or death. For stroke, estimates of relative risk reductions of beta-blockers compared to placebo ranged from 0 to 0.41.[7, 8, 10]

We found beta-blockers were a heterogeneous class of agents with various cardioselective actions and intrinsic sympathomimetic activity. We were unclear regarding whether cardiovascular benefits of different cardioselective beta-blockers represented a class effect.

ACE inhibitors

We did not find any large randomized trials with clinical outcomes that compared first-line therapy with an angiotensin converting enzyme (ACE) inhibitor to placebo in hypertensive people. We found a large, randomized placebo-controlled trial that showed an ACE inhibitor, ramipril, reduced cardiovascular events by 22% (relative risk 0.78; 95% CI 0.70 to 0.86) and death by 16% in high-risk people.[11](Tx: LIb) Approximately 50% of the trial participants had hypertension, approximately 50% had a history of myocardial infarction, and approximately 40% were taking beta-blockers. Participants with hypertension had relative risk reductions for cardiovascular events that were equal or greater than those observed among all participants.

We found data in hypertensive people were insufficient to judge whether any cardiovascular benefits of ACE inhibitors represented a class effect.

Calcium channel blockers

We found one large randomized trial that compared a long-acting dihydropyridine calcium channel blocker, nisoldipine, with placebo in people aged 60 and older with isolated systolic hypertension.[12](Tx: LIb) Rates of cardiovascular events with active treatment were reduced by 0.31 (95% CI 14% to 0.45%).

We found calcium channel blockers were a very heterogeneous class of agents with various postulated mechanisms of action. Data regarding harms associated with various calcium channel blockers are described below and in Chapter 6. Such data suggest that calcium channel blockers are unlikely to have class effects in hypertensive people.

Alpha-agonists and alpha-blockers

We did not find any large randomized trials with clinical outcomes that compared first-line therapy with either alpha-agonists, such as clonidine, or alpha-blockers, such as terazosin or doxazosin, with placebo.

Relative efficacy of different antihypertensive agents

ACE inhibitors versus diuretics and/or beta-blockers versus calcium channel blockers

We found an open, long-term trial, involving 6600 patients aged 70 to 84, that reported no differences in blood pressure control or cardiovascular morbidity or mortality among people randomized to conventional therapy with diuretics and/or beta-blockers versus calcium channel blockers (felodipine or isradipine) versus ACE inhibitors (enalapril or lisinopril).[13](Tx: LIb) We found a single-blind, long-term trial involving 10 985 patients aged 25 to 66 years that reported an ACE inhibitor (captopril) was not more effective than conventional therapy (diuretics or beta-blockers) in reducing cardiovascular morbidity or mortality.[14](Tx: L2b) We found the latter results inconclusive because a flaw in the randomization process resulted in unbalanced groups.

We found two additional smaller trials that compared either nisoldipine with enalapril or amlodipine with fosinopril in hypertensive patients with Type 2 diabetes.[15, 16](Tx: L2b) They found ACE inhibitors and calcium channel blockers were equally effective in reducing blood pressure, but calcium channel blockers were associated with a two- to five-fold increase in cardiovascular events compared to ACE inhibitors. We found one trial that compared captopril with atenolol in hypertensive patients with Type 2 diabetes.[17](Tx: LIb) There were no significant differences between groups in blood pressure levels or cardiovascular events. (See Chapter 6 for further discussion.)

Alpha-blockers versus diuretics

We found one randomized trial that found the alpha-blocker, doxazosin, increased cardiovascular events, particularly congestive heart failure, compared to a diuretic, chlorthalidone.[18](Tx: LIb)

Beta-blockers versus diuretics

We found five trials involving nearly 20 000 people that directly compared first-line therapy with thiazide diuretics with first-line therapy with beta-blockers.[8](Tx: LIa) Pooled data showed no statistically significant differences in cardiovascular outcomes (relative risk 0.88; 95% CI 0.78 to 1.00 thiazide versus beta-blocker) or death (relative risk 0.97; 95% CI 0.84 to 1.11). We found systematic reviews that compared results of trials that used diuretics as first-line agents with results of trials that used beta-blockers as first-line agents.[7-9] These showed no significant differences between diuretics and beta-blockers, although only diuretics showed significant reductions in coronary heart disease events.

Calcium channel blockers versus diuretics and beta-blockers

We found one double-blind randomized trial that compared a calcium channel blocker, long-acting nifedipine, with a combination thiazide-amiloride diuretic.[19](Tx: L2b) Participants were 6321 men and women with hypertension and at least one additional cardiovascular risk factor. No significant differences were reported between groups in cardiovascular events (relative risk 1.10; 95% CI 0.91 to 1.34 nifedipine versus diuretic). We found a second, large open randomized trial that compared diltiazem to diuretics and/or beta-blockers in over 10 000 Scandinavian men and women aged 50 to 74.[20](Tx: L1b) Initially a short-acting formulation of diltiazem was used; this was switched in the later years of the trial to a long-acting formulation. After four to five years, cardiovascular events were similar between groups (relative risk 1.0; 95% CI 0.87 to 1.15 diltiazem versus diuretic/beta-blocker).

Tolerability

We found recent studies of low-dose drugs showed good tolerance. For example, 72% of patients remained on their initially assigned treatment for four years, compared to 59% of people on placebo in a double-blind trial that compared placebo with five antihypertensive agents.[21]

We are unclear regarding which specific antihypertensive agents are most tolerable to patients. In all but one of four long-term, double-blind comparisons of low-dose diuretics, beta-blockers, ACE inhibitors, and calcium channel blockers, tolerability and overall quality of life indicators tended to be more favorable for diuretics and beta-blockers than for newer drugs.[19, 22-24](Tx: L1b) The exception showed fewer overall, but more serious effects with diuretics compared to nifedipine, a long-acting calcium channel blocker.[19](H: L1b) Serious effects were defined as "life-threatening, disabling, or leading to hospital admission." In drug-drug trials comparing thiazides with beta-blockers, thiazides were associated with significantly lower rates of withdrawal due to adverse effects (relative risk 0.69; 95% CI 4.2% to 7.2%).[8](H: L1a)

Drugs with bothersome harms

Symptomatic adverse effects vary by drug class and by agents within classes. For example, in a recent large trial of 6600 elders followed for five years, 26% of people receiving calcium channel blockers (felodipine or isradipine) report ankle edema, 30% receiving ACE inhibitors (enalapril or lisonopril) report cough, and 9% of people receiving diuretics and/or beta-blockers report cold hands and feet.[13] Although we do not discuss bothersome adverse effects related to specific agents in much detail, Chapter 6 provides additional information about adverse effects such as sexual dysfunction attributable to specific agents.

Drugs with possible major morbid or mortal harms

We found case-control, cohort, and randomized studies suggest that short and intermediate acting dihydropyridine calcium channel blockers, such as nifedipine and isradipine, may increase cardiovascular morbidity and mortality.[25](H: L1, L2, L3) A large trial suggests that an alpha-agonist, doxazosin, increases risk of cardiovascular events, particularly congestive heart failure compared to chlorthalidone.[18](H: L1b) One systematic review of nine case-control and three cohort studies has reported approximate two-fold increases in renal cell carcinoma risk with long-term diuretic use.[26] Absolute risks cannot be calculated from these studies, but are likely low as renal cell carcinoma is uncommon.

Our practiced judgments

We consider several agents appropriate options for initial treatment of hypertension (Table 4.3). Of the options, we routinely prefer thiazide diuretics as first-line therapy for hypertensive patients who do not have specific comorbid conditions that warrant particular treatment. (See Chapter 6 for a discussion of several comorbid conditions that warrant special treatment consideration.) We avoid alpha-agonists and short-acting calcium channel blockers.

Table 4.3. First-line antihypertensive drug options for people with hypertension.

Effective	Unclear	Possibly harmful
Thiazide diuretics	Angiotensin II receptor blockers	Alpha-agonists
Some beta-blockers	Some beta-blockers	Short-acting calcium channel blockers
ACE inhibitors	Some calcium channel blockers	
Some long-acting calcium channel blockers		

What are the benefits and harms of treating dyslipidemia in people with hypertension?

We found approximately a two-fold increase in the risk of cardiovascular disease in people with elevations in total and low-density lipoprotein (LDL) cholesterol and low levels of high-density lipoprotein (HDL) compared to people without such findings. We were unclear regarding whether elevated triglyceride levels conferred increased independent risk (see Chapter 3).

Benefits of drug treatment for individuals with elevated LDL and total cholesterol levels and/or decreased HDL levels

We found multiple randomized placebo-controlled trials that consistently showed treatment of elevated LDL and total cholesterol with diet and drug therapy reduced the five-year incidence of cardiovascular events and death by approximately 30% in middle-aged and older men and women (95% CI approximately 20% to 50%).[27-30](Tx: LIa) Risk reductions in myocardial infarction and coronary heart disease-related mortality occurred among people who had known cardiovascular disease (secondary prevention) as well as among those without known cardiovascular disease (primary prevention).[30](Tx: LIa) Risk reductions, which were apparent within one to two years of initiating drug treatment, increased with longer durations of treatment. Specifically, relative risk reductions were 7% (95% CI 0% to 14%) with two years of treatment, 22% (95% CI 15% to 28%) with two to five years of treatment, and 25% (95% CI 15% to 35%) with greater than five years of treatment.[31] We found that evidence was unclear regarding whether risk reductions continue to increase with treatment duration of greater than eight to ten years.

We found one large, double-blind, randomized trial that reported gemfibrozil, a fibrate, given for five years improved clinical outcomes in men with known coronary heart disease and low levels of HDL cholesterol (less than 1.0 mmol/L or 40 mg/dL).[32](Tx: LIb) Participants in this trial had LDL cholesterol levels that were 3.6 mmol/L (140 mg/dL) or less and average triglyceride levels of 1.8 mmol/L (160 mg/dL). Gemfibrozil increased HDL levels by 6% and decreased triglyceride levels by 31%. Relative risk reductions in morbid and mortal coronary heart disease events with treatment were 22% (95% CI 7% to 35%). Another randomized, placebo-controlled trial evaluated whether bezafibrate improved outcomes in people with previous myocardial infarction or stable angina and the following lipid profile: HDL below 45 mg/dL; triglyceride below 300 mg/dL, and LDL below 180 mg/dL.[33](Tx: L2b)

Compared to placebo, bezafibrate given for six years significantly reduced triglyceride levels by 21% and increased HDL levels by 18%, but did not significantly affect clinical cardiovascular outcomes. The trial had limited power to detect clinically important differences between groups and was confounded by people in both groups receiving a second active agent, colestipol.

Multiple trials suggested that individuals with greater baseline risk of future cardiovascular disease were more likely to personally benefit from drug therapy over five to ten years than were individuals with lower baseline risks.[27-30](Tx: IIa) However, we found evidence of clinical benefits of drug treatment for people without known cardiovascular disease, as long as they had a potential annual risk of coronary heart disease events of greater than 1% to 2%.[30](Tx: IIa) We found no clear threshold level whereby further lowering of cholesterol would result in either more harm than benefit or more benefit than harm.

We found no large long-term trials that directly compared the clinical effects of different drug therapies aimed at lowering cholesterol and/or increasing HDL. Across trials that have compared particular agents such as cholestyramine, gemfibrozil, or a statin with placebo, statins produced the largest reductions in cholesterol and the largest reductions in cardiovascular events.[30] Benefits of statins seemed to be fully explained by their lipid-lowering ability.

Benefits of diet treatment for individuals with elevated LDL and total cholesterol levels and/or decreased HDL levels

We found reviews of several randomized trials that evaluated effects of low-fat diet on cholesterol.[34,35](Tx: IIa) Modest sustained reductions of approximately 3% to 6% in total cholesterol over several months were reported. More intense low-fat diets appeared to result in greater reductions in cholesterol than less intense diets. We did not find any high quality, long-term trials that evaluated whether low-fat diets decreased the incidence of cardiovascular disease among people with dyslipidemia.

Benefits of treating people with elevated triglyceride levels

We found no large long-term randomized trials that evaluated whether treatment of isolated hypertriglyceridemia results in decreased cardiovascular disease.

Benefits of treating dyslipidemia in people with diabetes

We found one double-blind, randomized trial that evaluated clinical effects of bezafibrate in people with Type 2 diabetes and no known cardiovascular disease.[36](Tx: L2b) Participants had at least one of the following lipid parameters: total cholesterol at or above 5.2 mmol/L, triglyceride at or above 1.8 mmol/L, HDL at or below 1.1 mmol/L, or total cholesterol to HDL ratio at or above 4.7. Compared to placebo, bezafibrate significantly improved all lipid parameters and decreased coronary heart disease events (7% versus 23%).

We found one randomized trial that evaluated clinical effects of fenofibrate in people with Type 2 diabetes, mild dyslipidemia, and angiographically detectable stenosis.[37](Tx: L2b) Participants had dyslipidemia typically seen in people with diabetes: mean triglyceride 2.42 mmol/L, mean LDL 3.43 mmol/L, mean HDL 1.01 mmol/L, and total cholesterol to HDL ratio above 4. Compared to placebo, fenofibrate given for three years lowered total cholesterol and triglycerides by 30% and increased HDL levels by 8%. Fenofibrate significantly reduced progression of focal atherosclerotic lesions and decreased combined cardiovascular endpoints, such as cardiovascular death, myocardial infarction, bypass surgery, and hospitalizations by 23%. The latter comparison was not statistically significant.

Harms

We found no consistent evidence from randomized trials or large surveillance studies of frequent, serious, or life-threatening adverse effects of drug therapy for dyslipidemia.[35] Myopathy and muscle pain occur rarely in less than 1% of people taking statins.[35]

Our practiced judgments

We recommend diet and drug therapy for all of our patients who have hypertension, dyslipidemia (elevated LDL cholesterol or LDL below 3.6 mmol/L and decreased HDL), and known cardiovascular disease. In hypertensive people without known cardiovascular disease, we use risk equations, such as those described in Chapter 3, to estimate their individual future risk of cardiovascular disease. We recommend diet and drug therapy for those patients who have an estimated annual risk of coronary heart disease of greater than 1%. Most of our hypertensive patients have such risks. As of August 2000, we are generally reluctant to prescribe drug therapy for our hypertensive patients with isolated fasting hypertriglyceridemia, but we do discuss therapeutic options and their unknown but potential benefit and harm with people who have diabetes or very high levels of fasting triglycerides (greater than 7.9 mmol/L or 750 mg/dL).

What are the benefits and harms of smoking cessation in people with hypertension?

Smoking is strongly positively associated with increased overall mortality, coronary and cerebrovascular disease, various cancers, and respiratory disease.[38, 39](Pr: L1, L2, L3) For example, smokers are about three times more likely to die in middle age and twice as likely to die in older age (over age 65) compared with lifelong nonsmokers.[40,41](Pr: L1a) Greater amounts of tobacco use are associated with greater risks.

Benefits of quit-smoking strategies

We found several strategies, such as counseling and nicotine replacement, were effective in increasing quit rates among smokers.[38, 39](Tx: L1a) We found no randomized trials that evaluated whether quit-smoking advice and smoking cessation led to sustained reductions in blood pressure. Several large cohort studies suggested that smoking cessation reduced risk of cardiovascular disease, cancer, and respiratory disease.[38, 39](Tx: L2a)

Beneficial reductions in death rates with quitting smoking

In cohort studies, people who stopped smoking had death rates that fell gradually to lie between those of lifelong smokers and never smokers.[40,42](Tx: L2a) We found no precise estimates regarding the time required for former smokers to reduce their risk of death near the risk observed in never smokers, but above studies suggested that such risk reduction may take as long as a decade or more.

Beneficial reductions in coronary heart disease rates with quitting smoking

We found one large trial in middle-aged men that showed routine advice to quit smoking, compared with no routine advice, led to an average fall in cigarette consumption of 53% and to a corresponding statistically nonsignificant fall in the relative risk of death from coronary heart disease of 0.18 (95% CI −0.18 to 0.43).[43](Tx: L1c) We found cohort studies that suggested that the risk of coronary events is decreased when smokers quit smoking and that such risk declined to a level comparable to that of never smokers after two to three years.[38](Tx: L2) Declining risks were independent of the number of cigarettes smoked before quitting.

Beneficial reductions in stroke rates with quitting smoking

We found multiple observational studies that reported the risk of stroke decreased in ex-smokers compared with smokers.[38](Tx: L2a) We found variable estimates, ranging from two to ten years, regarding how long it took to reduce risk of stroke to levels of nonsmokers.[38, 41, 44]

Harms

We found no evidence that stopping smoking increases serious or life-threatening events or death.

Our practiced judgments

We routinely advise our hypertensive patients who are smoking to quit, and we refer them to various clinic and community counseling and nicotine replacement programs. We also routinely advise our hypertensive patients who are not presently smoking to avoid tobacco.

What are the benefits and harms of routine physical activity in people with hypertension?

Benefits

Normotensive and hypertensive people who are physically active and physically fit typically have one-fifth to one-half of the relative risk of coronary heart disease and stroke, compared with people who are sedentary or physically unfit.[34, 45](Pr: L1, L2, L3) Risk of cardiovascular disease declines with increasing levels of activity. In absolute terms, people leading sedentary lives (those who never or rarely engaged in any physical activity) suffered about 70 cardiovascular heart disease deaths per 10 000 person years compared with 40 per 10 000 person years among the most active participants (those who expend over 3500 kcal per week). This translates to an estimated benefit from high levels of physical activity of about 30 lives saved per 10 000 person years at risk.[34]

We found no randomized trials that examined the effects of long-term physical activity on morbidity, mortality, or quality of life. Multiple trials showed exercise interventions, such as walking/jogging, cycling, or both, often lasting 45 to 60 minutes per session, for three days per week reduced blood pressure.[46, 47](Tx: L1a) Compared with nonexercising control groups, aerobic exercise reduced systolic blood pressure by 4.7 mm Hg (95% CI 4.4

to 5.0 mm Hg) and diastolic blood pressure by 3.1 mm Hg (95% CI 3.0 to 3.3 mm Hg).[46] Greater reductions were seen in people with higher initial blood pressures. Trials in hypertensive adults that tested long-term exercise programs of greater than six months' duration found variable, insignificant mean reductions in systolic blood pressure (systolic reduction 0.8 mm Hg; 95% CI 5.9 mm Hg reduction to 4.2 mm Hg increase).[47](Tx: L1)

Several small, randomized controlled trials of varying quality suggest that at least moderate-intensity exercise (equivalent to brisk walking) over six to 12 months is necessary to improve fitness and increase maximal oxygen consumption. We found no conclusive evidence regarding differences of benefits between short bouts of exercise several times a day compared with longer daily bouts. The type and amount of exercise most likely to result in cardiovascular benefits are unclear, with some recent studies showing some benefits with simple increases in lifestyle activity. For example, a cohort study involving 173 hypertensive men has shown "regular heavy activity several times weekly" compared to no or limited spare time physical activity reduced all-cause (relative risk 0.43; 95% CI 0.22 to 0.82) and cardiovascular mortality (relative risk 0.33; 95% CI 0.11 to 0.94).[45](Tx: L2b)

Harms

Musculoskeletal strains, sprains, and injuries are the most likely adverse effects of physical activity. We did not find any representative population-based studies that characterized the exact type and frequency of injuries likely to occur with physical activity; these are likely to vary depending upon the nature of the chosen physical activity.

The absolute risk of sudden death after strenuous activity is small; it has been variously estimated at six deaths per 100 000 middle-aged men per year or 0.3 to 2.7 events per 10 000 person hours of exercise.[48] Risk of sudden death is greatest among people who have been previously habitually sedentary.[48-52] Specifically, strenuous activity is estimated to raise the relative risk of myocardial infarction between two and sixfold in the hour after activity, with risks returning to baseline after that. Risks appear much higher in people who are habitually sedentary (relative risk 107; 95% CI 67 to 171) compared with those who engaged in heavy physical exertion on five or more occasions per week (relative risk 2.4; 95% CI 1.5 to 3.7).[49] Injury is likely to be the most common adverse event, but few population data are available to quantify the magnitude of risk.

Our practiced judgments

Although the clinical significance of reductions in blood pressure observed with regular exercise is uncertain, regular physical activity is associated with decreased risk of cardiovascular disease. We routinely advise adults to maintain active lifestyles. As many adults may find regular exercise programs difficult to sustain, we repeat such advice at multiple visits and reinforce maintenance of physical activity for patients who are engaging in active lifestyles. As risks of sudden death are highest among habitually sedentary people, we recommend gradual programs of increasing exercise for people who are sedentary.

 # What are the benefits and harms of particular dietary interventions in people with hypertension?

Benefits of low-fat, high-fruit and vegetable diets

We found no randomized trials examining the effects of low-fat, high-fruit and vegetable diet on morbidity or mortality in people without known coronary disease. Multiple cohort studies have found that eating more fruit and vegetables is associated with decreased risk of heart attack and, possibly, stroke.[34, 53-55](Tx: L2) We found that the size of any real protective effect was uncertain.

We found data concerning low-fat diets were mixed in people with known cardiovascular disease. Moreover, systematic reviews and a large trial showed that low-fat diets compared to other control diets may or may not reduce death rates from coronary heart disease in people who have had a myocardial infarction.[56, 57](Tx: L2b) In the trial, reported relative risks of death among people assigned low-fat diets compared to controls was 0.95 (95% CI 0.75 to 1.27).[57]

We found one short trial involving 459 adults that showed a low-fat, high-fruit and vegetable diet modestly reduced blood pressure.[58](Tx: L2b) Participants had systolic blood pressures of below 160 mm Hg and diastolic blood pressures of 80 to 90 mm Hg. Food was provided to participants as one of three diets: a control diet low in magnesium and potassium; a fruit and vegetable diet high in potassium, magnesium, and fiber; and a combination of the fruit and vegetable diet with a low-fat diet high in calcium and protein. After eight weeks, the fruit and vegetable diet compared to the control diet reduced systolic blood pressure by 2.8 mm Hg (95% CI 0.9 to 4.7 mm Hg) and diastolic blood pressure by 1.1 mm Hg (95% CI 2.4 mm Hg decrease to 0.3 mm Hg increase). The combination diet compared to the control diet reduced systolic blood pressure by 5.5 mm Hg (95 % CI 3.7 to 7.4) and diastolic blood pressure by 3.0 mm Hg (95% CI 1.6 to 4.3).

Benefits of high-fish diets

We found no large randomized trials that evaluated whether high-fish diets improve survival in people without known cardiovascular disease. We found one large randomized trial that evaluated whether high-fish diets improve survival among people who have suffered a myocardial infarction.[57](Tx: IIb) The trial compared low-fat diet advice with high-fiber diet advice with high-fish diet advice of consuming at least two portions of fatty fish weekly. People given fish advice consumed three times the amount of fish compared to people not given such advice and were significantly less likely to die within two years (relative risk reduction 29%; 95% CI 7% to 40%). (For information related to fish oil consumption, see section on supplements.)

Benefits of Mediterranean diets

We found no large randomized trials that evaluated whether Mediterranean diets improve survival in people without known cardiovascular disease. We found one large randomized trial that compared "usual" dietary advice to advice to consume a Mediterranean-type diet in middle-aged people who had experienced a recent myocardial infarction.[59](Tx: IIb) The Mediterranean diet consisted of more bread, fruit, vegetables and fish, less meat, and replacement of butter and cream with rapeseed oil. This trial was stopped prematurely after two years because many fewer deaths were observed with the Mediterranean compared to the usual diet (relative risk reduction 70%; 95% CI 18% to 89%).

Benefits of salt restriction

We found multiple randomized trials that suggested, compared to usual diets, low-salt diets with or without weight reduction may modestly reduce blood pressure levels.[60, 61](Tx: IIa) We found trials that suggested people older than 45 years may have greater reductions in blood pressure than younger people and that lesser reductions in salt restriction (60 mmol daily) were less effective than higher reductions.[60-62] Actual salt intake in most of the trials was heterogeneous, but a mean reduction in sodium intake of 118 mmol (6.7 g) daily for 28 days led to reductions of 3.9 mm Hg (95% CI 3.0 to 4.8 mm Hg) in systolic blood pressure and 1.9 mm Hg (95% CI 1.3 to 2.5 mm Hg) in diastolic blood pressure.[60] In elderly people, one trial showed a mean decrease in salt intake of about 40 mmol (2.35 g) daily reduced systolic blood pressure by 2.6 mm Hg (95% CI 0.4 to 4.8 mm Hg) and diastolic blood pressure by 1.1 mm Hg (95% CI 0.3 mm Hg rise in diastolic to 2.5 mm Hg fall).[61] We found that small trials tended to report larger reductions in systolic and diastolic blood pressure than larger trials, which is consistent with publication bias or less rigorous methodology in small trials. We found no trials that examined the effects of salt restriction on morbidity or mortality.

Harms

We found no direct evidence that showed low-fat, high-fish, high-fruit and vegetable, or low-salt diets increase serious or life-threatening events or death. Epidemiological data regarding low-salt diets conflict, with one observational study suggesting that very low-salt intakes may be associated with increased incidence of myocardial infarction in middle-aged men.[63] Our experience is that the relative inconvenience and cost of various diets are likely to vary from person to person, depending upon prior diet and accessibility to particular foods.

Our practiced judgments

Multiple trials show that long-term maintenance of particular diets is difficult for many people. Although low-fat diets and low-salt diets both may have multiple benefits, we think the size and nature of their benefits are unclear, and we do not know whether their benefits accrue independently or are closely tied to other factors, such as socioeconomic status and physically active lifestyles.[34] Mediterranean-type diets high in fish, vegetables, and fruits and low in meat and butter appear to improve clinical outcomes in people who have had a myocardial infarction. Based on above data, we routinely encourage adults with hypertension to avoid high fat diets and to eat fish, fruits, and vegetables, but we do not routinely refer such patients for extensive dietary or nutrition counseling.

 # What are the benefits and harms of weight loss for hypertensive overweight patients?

Benefits

We found no randomized trials that examined the effects of weight loss on morbidity and mortality. We found multiple trials that showed modest weight reductions of 3% to 9% of body weight are achievable in motivated middle-aged and older adults and may lead to modest reductions in blood pressure in obese people with hypertension.[64](Tx: IIa) Participants in these trials had caloric intakes that ranged from 450 to 1500 kcal daily. Combined data from six trials that did not vary antihypertensive regimens during the weight loss intervention period showed mean blood pressure reductions of 3 mm Hg systolic (95% CI 0.7 to 6.8 mm Hg) and 2.9 mm Hg diastolic (95% CI 0.1 to 5.7 mm Hg). Trials that allowed adjustment of antihypertensive regimens found that lower doses and fewer antihypertensive drugs were needed in the weight reduction groups compared with control groups.

Harms

We found no direct evidence that intentional gradual weight loss of less than 10% of body weight was harmful.

Our practiced judgments

Although we find many adults find it difficult to achieve and maintain weight loss, we routinely recommend slow gradual weight loss in people who are overweight.

 # What are the benefits and harms of antiplatelet treatment in people with hypertension?

Benefits

We found four large randomized trials that evaluated whether aspirin chemoprophylaxis reduced the risk of coronary heart disease in people who were at low risk for cardiovascular disease (primary prevention).[65](Tx: LIa) Low-risk people were those who had a 1% to 7% five-year risk of cardiovascular disease. Three of the four trials used placebo controls and were conducted under double-blind conditions. Aspirin chemoprophylaxis was 500 mg daily or less in all the trials and was 75 mg daily in one. Pooled data showed aspirin chemoprophylaxis reduced fatal and nonfatal coronary heart disease by 28% (95% CI 11% to 41%). Overall, the incidence of stroke (summary odds ratio 1.06; 95% CI 0.89 to 1.26) and death (summary odds ratio 0.94; 95% CI 0.85 to 1.04) were not affected.

We found that two of the trials reported cardiovascular risk reductions among patients with hypertension.[66,67] However, a subanalysis of one of the trials suggested aspirin reduced cardiovascular events in patients with systolic blood pressure levels of 130 to 145 mm Hg (relative risk 0.68) but not in patients with systolic pressures greater than 145 mm Hg (relative risk 1.08).[68]

We expect additional important information soon will become available from the women's health study, a randomized trial that is comparing aspirin 100 mg daily versus placebo among 40 000 healthy postmenopausal women.[69]

We found multiple randomized trials that evaluated whether aspirin reduced cardiovascular events in people with high-risk or known cardiovascular disease.[34, 70](Tx: LIa) Compared to placebo, aspirin reduced the odds of a cardiovascular event by approximately 25% (summary odds reduction 27%; 95% CI 24% to 30%).[70] Trials that directly compared various doses of aspirin generally reported similar efficacy with 75 to 325 mg daily doses compared to higher 500 to 1500 mg daily doses.

We found randomized placebo-controlled trials that showed thienopyridine agents, such as clopidogrel or ticlopidine also are effective in reducing cardiovascular events in people with high risk or known cardiovascular disease.[34, 70] We found data comparing aspirin with thienopyridine agents were scarce. One large randomized trial directly compared aspirin and clopidogrel in several thousand people with recent stroke or myocardial infarction or peripheral vascular disease.[71](Tx: IIb) Clopidogrel reduced cardiovascular events slightly more than aspirin (relative risk reduction 8.7%; 95% CI 0.3% to 16.5%).

Harms

We found several pooled analyses from multiple randomized trials that showed aspirin prophylaxis increases odds of gastrointestinal bleeding by approximately 1.5 to twofold. [72-74](H: IIa) Increased risks were found with low-dose prophylaxis consisting of 75 to 325 mg daily as well as for higher doses of aspirin.[75, 76] We found evidence was unclear regarding whether higher doses were associated with marked increased risk of bleeding.[75-77] Risks did not appear lower with enteric-coated or buffered preparations, and concomitant use of nonsteroidal antiinflammatory agents or anticoagulants increased risks.

We found aspirin was associated with a small increased risk of hemorrhagic stroke, but most available evidence was derived from middle-aged men and may not apply to elders who have higher baseline rates of both ischemic and hemorrhagic stroke.

Our practiced judgments

We have modeled estimated benefits and harms of aspirin prophylaxis for patients with various levels of baseline risks for cardiovascular disease (Table 4.4).[65] We routinely advise hypertensive patients with known cardiovascular disease, as well as patients with high risks for a future cardiovascular event, that aspirin prophylaxis is more likely to benefit than harm them. We consider patients to be high-risk when their estimated five-year risks of cardiovascular events are 5% or greater. We advise patients that the main potential benefits of aspirin prophylaxis are prevention of heart attacks and that the main potential harms are gastrointestinal bleeds and, to a lesser extent, hemorrhagic strokes. We routinely advise clopidogrel for patients with known cardiovascular disease who cannot take aspirin.

Table 4.4. Estimation of benefits and harms of low-dose aspirin for people with various levels of baseline risk for cardiovascular events*.

Benefits and harms	Baseline risk over five years			
	1%	3%	5%	10%
Effect on total mortality	No effect	No effect	No effect	Possible small reduction
CVD events** avoided in aspirin-treated	3	8	14	28
Effect on ischemic stroke	No change?	No change?	No change?	1 to 3 prevented
Excess hemorrhagic strokes in aspirin-treated	1 to 2	1 to 2	1 to 2	1 to 2
Excess major gastrointestinal bleeds in aspirin-treated	3 to 7	3 to 7	3 to 7	3 to 7

*Estimates are based on 1000 patients receiving aspirin for five years and a relative risk reduction of 28% for cardiovascular events with aspirin.

**CVD events include nonfatal acute myocardial infarction and fatal coronary heart disease.

What are the benefits and harms of modest alcohol consumption in people with hypertension?

Benefits

We found that observational studies consistently showed an inverse relationship between coronary artery disease and alcohol consumption.[78] However, consuming more than two drinks daily (approximately 20g of ethanol) was associated with increased total mortality, due primarily to increased incidence of cancer, trauma, and cirrhosis.[79](Pr: L1, L2) We found numerous population studies that reported positive associations between higher alcohol consumption and higher blood pressure levels; the relation was generally linear, although several studies reported a threshold effect at around two to three standard drinks a day.[80]

We found a systematic review of seven trials involving 751 hypertensive people randomized to decrease or quit drinking versus no such advice. Data were inconclusive regarding blood pressure benefits of alcohol reduction among moderate to heavy drinkers (25 to 50 drinks weekly).[81] Substantial reductions in alcohol use in both control and intervention groups limited ability to detect differences between groups.

Harms

We found no direct evidence that reducing alcohol intake to as few as two drinks a day is harmful. Multiple studies show higher intakes are positively associated with higher death, cancer, trauma, and cirrhosis rates.

Our practiced judgments

We routinely advise our hypertensive patients who do not have a history of substance abuse that consuming one to two drinks per day is probably safe and possibly protective, but that more than this is likely harmful. We routinely advise patients with histories of substance abuse not to consume alcohol.

 # What are the benefits and harms of anticoagulant treatment in people with hypertension?

Benefits

We found one large placebo-controlled trial that evaluated whether oral anticoagulation with low-dose warfarin or aspirin improves clinical outcomes in individuals without evidence of cardiovascular disease.[82] The targeted international normalized ratio (INR) for patients assigned to warfarin was 1.5. Compared with placebo, warfarin reduced the rate of all coronary heart disease by 21% (95% CI 4% to 35%) and had no statistically significant effect on the rate of strokes or cardiovascular death.

We found multiple randomized controlled trials that evaluated whether oral anticoagulation with warfarin improves clinical outcomes in people with known cardiovascular disease.[83](Tx: LIa) Pooled analyses showed that high intensity anticoagulation with target aims of INR greater than 2.8 decreased the odds of death, stroke and myocardial infarction by 43% (95% CI 37% to 49%). Moderate-intensity anticoagulation with a target INR within the 2.0 to 3.0 range did not significantly decrease the odds of death, stroke, and myocardial infarction. Trials that directly compared moderate- or high-intensity oral anticoagulation with aspirin showed similar effects of these agents on death, myocardial infarction, and stroke. Pooled analyses of trials that evaluated combination regimens of oral anticoagulation added to aspirin were inconclusive. However, they suggested low-intensity warfarin with target INR less than 1.5 added to warfarin was not significantly superior to aspirin alone in decreasing death, myocardial infarction, and stroke (odds ratio 0.91, 95% 0.79 to 1.06).

Harms

We found that pooled analyses of multiple, randomized controlled trials showed moderate- to high-intensity oral anticoagulation compared to control increased the odds of major bleeds approximately six- to eightfold. Most of these bleeds were gastrointestinal and extracranial. Pooled analyses show high- or moderate-intensity oral anticoagulation compared to aspirin increases odds of major bleeds by more than twofold (odds ratio 2.4; 95% CI 1.6 to 3.6).[83](H: LIa)

Our practiced judgments

We routinely advise our hypertensive patients to take aspirin rather than warfarin.

What are the benefits and harms of various antioxidants and vitamins for people with hypertension?

Antioxidant minerals

We found little evidence that either supported or refuted cardio-protective associations of copper, zinc, or manganese.[84] Cohort studies, carried out primarily in Finland where intake of selenium is low, report increased risk of ischemic heart disease in people with low blood selenium concentrations.[85](Pr: LIb)

Beta-Carotene

Prospective cohort studies of ß-carotene report protective associations between increased intake of ß-carotene and cardiovascular disease.[86–88](Pr: LIa) However, large trials do not show benefits and suggest harm.[89–91](Tx: L2b) For example, one trial suggests supplements are associated with a relative risk increase for cardiovascular deaths of 0.12 (95% CI 0.04 to 0.22).[91] Whether the trial findings are specific to a particular isomer or dose of ß-carotene is not clear.

Vitamin C

Multiple cohort studies have shown variable results regarding associations between vitamin C and coronary heart disease and stroke.[86, 89] (Pr: L2) We found no large, long-term trials that evaluated clinical effects of vitamin C supplementation.

Vitamin E

Multiple large cohort studies show positive associations between increased dietary or supplemental vitamin E intake and ischemic heart disease.[86, 92–95](Pr: L1b, L2b) Four large randomized controlled trials have evaluated clinical benefits of vitamin E.[91, 96–98](Tx: L1b) The largest trial included 29133 male Finnish smokers with and without known cardiovascular disease.[91] Other trials were limited primarily to participants with known cardiovascular disease. Daily doses that have been evaluated are 30 mg, 300 mg, 400 IU, and 800 IU (1 IU=0.67 mg). The individual trials have reported mixed results; decreases in nonfatal coronary heart disease events, as well as increases in coronary heart disease death, have been suggested. Pooled analyses of the trials showed no evidence that vitamin E affected cardiovascular disease incidence or death.[34]

Multivitamins

A large factorial trial from China has compared combinations of the following: retinol (10000 IU) and zinc (22.5 mg); riboflavin (5.2 mg) and niacin (40 mg); ascorbic acid (120 mg) and molybdenum (30 µg); and ß-carotene (15 mg), selenium (50 µg), and vitamin E (30 mg).[34](Tx: L2b) After six years, the combination of ß-carotene, selenium, and vitamin E showed a relative risk reduction in death from all causes of 0.09 (95% CI 0.01 to 0.16). Other combinations were not associated with reductions in stroke or death. A second trial from China randomized people with esophageal dysplasia to receive a multivitamin supplement that contained 14 vitamins and 12 minerals. The supplement included vitamin C (180 mg), vitamin E (60 IU), ß-carotene (15 mg), and selenium (50 µg). After six years, the relative risk reduction for death was 0.07 (95% CI 0.16 relative risk increase to 0.25 relative risk reduction) and for stroke was 0.33 (95% CI 0.07 relative risk increase to 0.63 relative risk reduction).[99, 100](Tx: L2b)

Fish oil

Several short-term trials of a few months in duration have found that fish oil (omega-3 polyunsaturated fatty acids) supplementation in large doses of greater than or equal to 3g daily modestly lowers blood pressure.[101](Tx: L2b) The mean decrease in blood pressure in the treatment groups relative to the control groups was approximately 4.5 mm Hg systolic (95% CI 1.2 to 7.8 mm Hg) and 2.5 mm Hg diastolic (95% CI 0.6 to 4.4 mm Hg). We found no evidence of beneficial effect on blood pressure at lower intakes of less than 3g daily. Belching, bad breath, fishy taste, and/or abdominal pain occur in about one-third of people taking high doses of fish oil.

We found no trials that examined effects of fish oil supplementation on morbidity and mortality in people without known cardiovascular disease. We found one large randomized trial that showed people who had survived a myocardial infarction who were assigned to receive 1 g daily of fish oil versus no fish oil were less likely to die within three to four years (relative risk reduction 0.14; 95% CI 0.03 to 0.24).[96](Tx: LIb)

Flavonoids

Multiple cohort studies report variable associations between increased flavonoid intake and ischemic heart disease.[55, 102–105](Pr: L2, L3) One observational study reported a reduced risk of stroke with increased flavonoid intake.[106](Tx: L4)

Our practiced judgments

We routinely advise our hypertensive patients to avoid β-carotene, and the benefits of vitamins and supplements other than fish oil are likely nonexistent or small. We do tell people with past myocardial infarctions that fish oil supplements may improve survival.

 # What are the benefits and harms of garlic, potassium, calcium, and magnesium supplementation in people with hypertension?

Benefits

We found no verifiable randomized trials that examined the effects of garlic, potassium, calcium, or magnesium supplementation on morbidity or mortality. We found 30 trials that measured blood pressure outcomes among people randomized to garlic supplementation compared to placebo or nonplacebo controls.[107](Tx: L2b) Garlic preparations that were used varied widely, biologically active constituents of studied preparations were often unclear, blinding of participants and observers was often suspect, and cointerventions with antihypertensive therapies were often not described. Although several trials reported within group significant reductions in blood pressure, only three demonstrated statistically significant reductions in blood pressure between people randomized to garlic and those serving as controls.

We found several trials that showed that daily potassium supplementation of about 60 mmol (2000 mg, which is roughly the amount contained in five bananas) reduces blood pressure a little.[108](Tx: LIa, LIb, L2b) Interventions most often consisted of potassium chloride supplementation ranging from 60 to 100 mmol daily. The mean decrease in blood pressure in the intervention groups compared with controls was 4.4 mm Hg systolic (95% CI 2.2 to 6.6 mm Hg) and 2.5 mm Hg diastolic (95% CI 0.1 to 4.9 mm Hg).

Several short-term, small randomized trials of several weeks duration in normotensive and hypertensive adults showed calcium supplementation ranging from 500 to 2000 mg daily may reduce systolic blood pressure by very small amounts.[109](Tx: L2b) On average, mean systolic blood pressure reduction was 1.4 mm Hg (95% CI 0.7 to 2.2 mm Hg); mean diastolic reduction was 0.8 (95% CI 0.2 to 1.4 mm Hg). We found no good evidence on the effect of magnesium supplementation on blood pressure in people with hypertension and normal magnesium concentrations; a few small, short-term trials have reported mixed results.[34](Tx: L2b)

Harms

We found most garlic supplements are associated with malodorous breath and body odor (H: L1a) and possibly esophageal or abdominal pain, flatulence, and bleeding.[107](H: L2b, L4) We found no direct evidence of harm from potassium supplementation in people without kidney failure and in people not taking drugs that increase serum potassium. We found gastrointestinal adverse effects, such as belching, flatulence, diarrhea, or abdominal discomfort, can occur in as many as 10% of people taking potassium supplements. We found reported adverse gastrointestinal effects of calcium supplementation, such as abdominal pain, were generally mild and varied among particular preparations.

Our practiced judgments

We routinely advise our hypertensive patients that the cardiovascular benefits of taking supplements, such as garlic, potassium, calcium, or magnesium, are unknown but likely to be small or nonexistent.

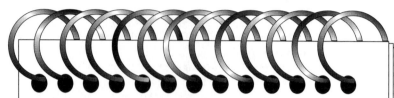

Patient Notes

Mr Willie Maykit

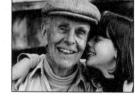

- Hypertensive diabetic
- On multiple medications and supplements

Actions

- Continue metformin, ACE inhibitor, and aspirin.
- Advise discontinuation of ß-carotene.
- Advise little likely benefit of his supplements, such as magnesium, on blood pressure control or cardiovascular outcomes.
- Advise healthy high vegetable and fish diet, and regular physical activity.
- Check lipid levels.

Summary bottom lines ▮▮▮▮▮▮▮▮▮▮▮▮▮▮▮▮▮▮▮▮▮

- **Antihypertensive agents**. Inform patients that there are several appropriate options for initial treatment of hypertension (Table 4.3). Of the drug options, thiazide diuretics are well-proven, first-line agents for hypertensive patients without special comorbid conditions. Alternative agents with some albeit less proven evidence of efficacy are some beta-blockers, ACE inhibitors, and some long-acting calcium channel blockers. Avoid short-acting alpha-agonists and short-acting calcium channel blockers. (Level 1 evidence)

- **Dyslipidemia treatment**. Recommend diet and drug therapy for hypertensive patients with dyslipidemia (elevated LDL cholesterol or LDL less than 3.6 mmol/L and decreased HDL) and known cardiovascular disease. In hypertensive people without known cardiovascular disease, use risk equations such as those described in Chapter 3 to estimate their individual future risk of cardiovascular disease. Use diet and drug therapy in patients who have an estimated annual risk of coronary heart disease of greater than 1%. (Level 1 evidence)

- **Quit smoking advice**. Routinely advise hypertensive patients who smoke to quit. Refer people who are contemplating quitting to various clinic and community counseling, and nicotine replacement programs. Routinely advise hypertensive patients who do not smoke to avoid tobacco. (Level 1 evidence)

- **Regular physical activity**. Routinely advise adults to maintain active lifestyles. Although the clinical significance of reductions in blood pressure observed with regular exercise is uncertain, regular physical activity is associated with decreased risk of cardiovascular disease. As many adults may find regular exercise programs difficult to sustain, repeat advice at multiple visits and reinforce maintenance of physical activity for patients who are engaging in active lifestyles. As risks of sudden death are highest among habitually sedentary people, recommend gradual programs of increasing exercise for people who are sedentary. (Consensus opinion and Level 1 prognostic evidence)

- **Diet advice**. Maintenance of particular diets is difficult for many people. Inform patients that low-fat diets and low-salt diets both may have benefits, but the size and nature of their benefits are unclear. Do advise Mediterranean-type diets high in fish, vegetables, and fruits and low in meat and butter, particularly in people with known coronary heart disease, as this diet may improve clinical outcomes. (Level 1 evidence)

- **Weight loss advice**. Although many adults find it difficult to achieve and maintain weight loss, routinely recommend slow gradual weight loss in people who are overweight. (Consensus opinion)

- **Anticoagulant advice**. Consider aspirin rather than anticoagulant therapy for patients with known cardiovascular disease. Although anticoagulant therapy with warfarin likely will improve cardiovascular outcomes in such patients, realize it requires more intensive monitoring and is associated with higher incidences of major bleeds than aspirin. (Level 1 evidence)

- **Aspirin prophylaxis**. Advise hypertensive patients with known cardiovascular disease, as well as patients with high risks for a future cardiovascular event, that aspirin prophylaxis is more likely to benefit than harm them. Consider patients with estimated five-year risks of cardiovascular events that are 5% or greater to be high risk. Advise patients that the main potential benefits of aspirin prophylaxis are prevention of heart attacks and that the main potential harms are gastrointestinal bleeds and, to a lesser extent, hemorrhagic strokes. Advise clopidogrel for patients with known cardiovascular disease who cannot take aspirin. (Level 1 evidence)

- **Alcohol consumption**. Advise hypertensive patients who do not have a history of substance abuse that consuming one to two drinks per day is probably safe and possibly protective, but that more than this is likely harmful. Advise patients with histories of substance abuse not to consume alcohol. (Level 1 prognostic evidence)

- **Beta-carotene, vitamins, and fish oil**. Advise hypertensive patients to avoid supplements containing ß-carotene. Advise them that the benefits of vitamins and supplements other than fish oil are likely nonexistent or small. Do tell people with past myocardial infarctions that fish oil supplements may improve survival. (Mixed Level 1 evidence)

- **Garlic, calcium, potassium, and magnesium supplements**. Advise hypertensive patients that the cardiovascular benefits of taking supplements such as garlic, potassium, calcium, or magnesium are unknown but likely small or nonexistent. (Mixed Level 1 evidence)

We identified English language and human-related literature for this chapter by searching MEDLINE, the Cochrane Controlled Trial Registry, and PsycINFO. We searched for systematic reviews and meta-analyses addressing treatment of hypertension from 1966 to 2000. As there are more than 10000 randomized trials that address treatment of hypertension, we only searched for new trial evidence published since 1995. We screened titles/abstracts of approximately 500 systematic reviews and meta-analyses and approximately 1500 trials to help identify the highest quality relevant information to include in the chapter.

References

1. Gueyffier F, Froment A, Gouton M. New meta-analysis of treatment trials of hypertension: improving the estimate of therapeutic benefit. *J Hum Hypertens* 1996; **10**:1-8.

2. Quan A, Kerlikowske K, Gueyffier F, Boissel JP. Efficacy of treating hypertension in women. *J Gen Intern Med* 1999; **14**:718-29.

3. Beto JA, Bansal VK. Quality of life in treatment of hypertension. A metaanalysis of clinical trials. *Am J Hypertens* 1992; **5**:125-33.

4. Croog SH, Levine S, Testa MA, *et al*. The effects of antihypertensive therapy on the quality of life. *N Engl J Med* 1986; **314**:1657-64.

5. Mulrow CD, Cornell JA, Herrera CR, Kadri A, Farnett L, Aguilar C. Hypertension in the elderly. Implications and generalizability of randomized trials. *JAMA* 1994; **272**:1932-8.

6. Wright JM. Choosing a first-line drug in the management of elevated blood pressure: what is the evidence? 1: Thiazide diuretics. *CMAJ* 2000; **163**:57-60.

7. Psaty BM, Smith NL, Siscovick DS, *et al*. Health outcomes associated with antihypertensive therapies used as first-line agents. A systematic review and meta-analysis. *JAMA* 1997; **277**:739-45.

8. Wright JM, Lee CH, Chambers GK. Systematic review of antihypertensive therapies: does the evidence assist in choosing a first-line drug? *CMAJ* 1999; **161**:25-32.

9. Messerli FH, Grossman E, Goldbourt U. Are beta-blockers efficacious as first-line therapy for hypertension in the elderly? A systematic review. *JAMA* 1998; **279**:1903-7.

10. Wright JM. Choosing a first-line drug in the management of elevated blood pressure: what is the evidence? 2: Beta-blockers. *CMAJ* 2000; **163**:188-92.

11. Yusuf S, Sleight P, Pogue J, Bosch J, Davies R, Dagenais G. Effects of an angiotensin-converting-enzyme inhibitor, ramipril, on cardiovascular events in high-risk patients. The Heart Outcomes Prevention Evaluation Study Investigators [published erratum appears in *N Engl J Med* 2000; **342**:748]. *N Engl J Med* 2000; **342**:145-53.

12. Staessen JA, Fagard R, Thijs L, *et al*. Randomised double-blind comparison of placebo and active treatment for older patients with isolated systolic hypertension. The Systolic Hypertension in Europe (Syst-Eur) Trial Investigators. *Lancet* 1997; **350**:757-64.

13. Hansson L, Lindholm LH, Ekbom T, *et al*. Randomised trial of old and new antihypertensive drugs in elderly patients: cardiovascular mortality and morbidity: the Swedish Trial in Old Patients with Hypertension-2 study. *Lancet* 1999; **354**:1751-6.

14. Hansson L, Lindholm LH, Niskanen L, *et al*. Effect of angiotensin-converting-enzyme inhibition compared with conventional therapy on cardiovascular morbidity and mortality in hypertension: the Captopril Prevention Project (CAPPP) randomised trial. *Lancet* 1999; **353**:611-16.

15. Tatti P, Pahor M, Byington RP, *et al*. Outcome results of the Fosinopril Versus Amlodipine Cardiovascular Events Randomized Trial (FACET) in patients with hypertension and NIDDM. *Diabetes Care* 1998; **21**:597-603.

16. Estacio RO, Jeffers BW, Hiatt WR, Biggerstaff SL, Gifford N, Schrier RW. The effect of nisoldipine as compared with enalapril on cardiovascular outcomes in patients with non-insulin-dependent diabetes and hypertension. *N Engl J Med* 1998; **338**:645-52.

17. UK Prospective Diabetes Study Group. Efficacy of atenolol and captopril in reducing risk of macrovascular and microvascular complications in type 2 diabetes: UKPDS 39. *BMJ* 1998; **317**:713-20.

18. ALLHAT Collaborative Research Group. Major cardiovascular events in hypertensive patients randomized to doxazosin vs chlorthalidone: the antihypertensive and lipid-lowering treatment to prevent heart attack trial (ALLHAT). *JAMA* 2000; **283**:1967-75.

19. Brown MJ, Palmer CR, Castaigne A, *et al*. Morbidity and mortality in patients randomised to double-blind treatment with a long-acting calcium-channel blocker or

diuretic in the International Nifedipine GITS study: intervention as a goal in hypertension treatment (INSIGHT). *Lancet* 2000; **356**:366-72.

20. Hansson L, Hedner T, Lund-Johansen P, *et al.* Randomised trial of effects of calcium antagonists compared with diuretics and beta-blockers on cardiovascular morbidity and mortality in hypertension: the Nordic Diltiazem (NORDIL) study. *Lancet* 2000; **356**:359-65.

21. Grimm RH Jr, Grandits GA, Cutler JA, *et al.* Relationships of quality-of-life measures to long-term lifestyle and drug treatment in the Treatment of Mild Hypertension Study. *Arch Intern Med* 1997; **157**:638-48.

22. Neaton JD, Grimm RH Jr, Prineas RJ, *et al.* Treatment of Mild Hypertension Study. Final results. Treatment of Mild Hypertension Study Research Group. *JAMA* 1993; **270**:713-24.

23. Materson BJ, Reda DJ, Cushman WC, *et al.* Single-drug therapy for hypertension in men. A comparison of six antihypertensive agents with placebo. The Department of Veterans Affairs Cooperative Study Group on Antihypertensive Agents [published erratum appears in *N Engl J Med* 1994 ;**330**:1689]. *N Engl J Med* 1993; **328**:914-21.

24. Philipp T, Anlauf M, Distler A, Holzgreve H, Michaelis J, Wellek S. Randomised, double blind, multicentre comparison of hydrochlorothiazide, atenolol, nitrendipine, and enalapril in antihypertensive treatment: results of the HANE study. HANE Trial Research Group. *BMJ* 1997; **315**:154-9.

25. Cutler JA. Calcium-channel blockers for hypertension—uncertainty continues. *N Engl J Med* 1998; **338**:679-81.

26. Grossman E, Messerli FH, Goldbourt U. Does diuretic therapy increase the risk of renal cell carcinoma? *Am J Cardiol* 1999; **83**:1090-3.

27. Katerndahl DA, Lawler WR. Variability in meta-analytic results concerning the value of cholesterol reduction in coronary heart disease: a meta-meta-analysis. *Am J Epidemiol* 1999; **149**:429-41.

28. Froom J, Froom P, Benjamin M, Benjamin BJ. Measurement and management of hyperlipidemia for the primary prevention of coronary heart disease. *J Am Board Fam Pract* 1998; **11**:12-22.

29. LaRosa JC, He J, Vupputuri S. Effect of statins on risk of coronary disease: a meta-analysis of randomized controlled trials. *JAMA* 1999; **282**:2340-6.

30. Pignone M, Phillips C, Mulrow C. Use of lipid lowering drugs for primary prevention of coronary heart disease: meta-analysis of randomised trials. *BMJ* 2000; **321**:983-6.

31. Law MR, Wald NJ, Thompson SG. By how much and how quickly does reduction in serum cholesterol concentration lower risk of ischaemic heart disease? *BMJ* 1994; **308**:367-72.

32. Rubins HB, Robins SJ, Collins D, *et al.* Gemfibrozil for the secondary prevention of coronary heart disease in men with low levels of high-density lipoprotein cholesterol. Veterans Affairs High-Density Lipoprotein Cholesterol Intervention Trial Study Group. *N Engl J Med* 1999; **341**:410-18.

33. BIP Study Group. Secondary prevention by raising HDL cholesterol and reducing triglycerides in patients with coronary artery disease: the Bezafibrate Infarction Prevention (BIP) study. *Circulation* 2000; **102**:21-7.

34. Cardiovascular disorders. In: *Clinical evidence: a compendium of the best available evidence for effective health care.* Issue 3 (June). London, England: BMJ Publishing Group, 2000: 1-154.

35. Pignone MP, Phillips CJ, Lannon C, *et al. Screening for lipid disorders: a systematic review for the US Preventive Services Task Force, 2000.* Agency for Healthcare Research and Quality contract no: 290-97-0011; project no. 6919-003.

36. Elkeles RS, Diamond JR, Poulter C, *et al.* Cardiovascular outcomes in type 2 diabetes. A double-blind placebo-controlled study of bezafibrate: the St. Mary's, Ealing, Northwick Park Diabetes Cardiovascular Disease Prevention (SENDCAP) Study. *Diabetes Care* 1998; **21**:641-8.

37. The Diabetes Atherosclerosis Intervention Study (DAIS). Presented at the XIIth International Symposium on Atherosclerosis, 2000 Jun 26; Stockholm, Sweden.

38. United States. Public Health Service. Office of the Surgeon General. *The health benefits of smoking cessation: a report of the Surgeon General.* Rockville (MD): U.S. Department of Health and Human Services, Center for Chronic Disease Prevention and Health Promotion, Office on Smoking and Health, 1990. DHHS publication; no. (CDC) 90-8416.

39. Royal College of Physicians of London. *Smoking and health now: a new report and summary on smoking and its effects on health.* London, England: Pittman Medical and Scientific Pub. Co, 1971.

40. Doll R, Peto R, Wheatley K, Gray R, Sutherland I. Mortality in relation to smoking: 40 years' observations on male British doctors. *BMJ* 1994; **309**:901-11.

41. Kawachi I, Colditz GA, Stampfer MJ, *et al.* Smoking cessation in relation to total mortality rates in women. A prospective cohort study. *Ann Intern Med* 1993; **119**:992-1000.

42. Rogot E, Murray JL. Smoking and causes of death among U.S. veterans: 16 years of observation. *Public Health Rep* 1980; **95**:213-22.

43. Rose G, Hamilton PJ, Colwell L, Shipley MJ. A randomised controlled trial of anti-smoking advice: 10-year results. *J Epidemiol Community Health* 1982; **36**:102-8.

44. Wannamethee SG, Shaper AG, Ebrahim S. History of parental death from stroke or heart trouble and the risk of stroke in middle-aged men. *Stroke* 1996; **27**:1492-8.

45. Engstrom G, Hedblad B, Janzon L. Hypertensive men who exercise regularly have lower rate of cardiovascular mortality. *J Hypertens* 1999; **17**:737-42.

46. Halbert JA, Silagy CA, Finucane P, Withers RT, Hamdorf PA, Andrews GR. The effectiveness of exercise training in lowering blood pressure: a meta-analysis of randomised controlled trials of 4 weeks or longer. *J Hum Hypertens* 1997; **11**:641-9.

47. Ebrahim S, Smith GD. Lowering blood pressure: a systematic review of sustained effects of non-pharmacological interventions. *J Public Health Med* 1998; **20**:441-8.

48. Oberman A. Exercise and the primary prevention of cardiovascular disease. *Am J Cardiol* 1985; **55**:10D-20D.

49. Mittleman MA, Maclure M, Tofler GH, Sherwood JB, Goldberg RJ, Muller JE. Triggering of acute myocardial infarction by heavy physical exertion. Protection against triggering by regular exertion. Determinants of Myocardial Infarction Onset Study Investigators. *N Engl J Med* 1993; **329**:1677-83.

50. Willich SN, Lewis M, Lowel H, Arntz HR, Schubert F, Schroder R. Physical exertion as a trigger of acute myocardial infarction. Triggers and Mechanisms of Myocardial Infarction Study Group. *N Engl J Med* 1993; **329**:1684-90.

51. Pate RR, Pratt M, Blair SN, *et al.* Physical activity and public health. A recommendation from the Centers for Disease Control and Prevention and the American College of Sports Medicine. *JAMA* 1995; **273**:402-7.

52. Thompson PD. The cardiovascular complications of vigorous physical activity. *Arch Intern Med* 1996; **156**:2297-302.

53. Ness AR, Powles JW. Fruit and vegetables, and cardiovascular disease: a review. *Int J Epidemiol* 1997; **26**:1-13.

54. Law MR, Morris JK. By how much does fruit and vegetable consumption reduce the risk of ischaemic heart disease? *Eur J Clin Nutr* 1998; **52**:549-56.

55. Klerk M, Jansen MCJF, Van't Veer P, Kok FJ. *Fruits and vegetables in chronic disease prevention.* Wageningen, Netherlands: Grafisch Bedrijf Ponsen and Looijen, 1998.

56. NHS Centre for Reviews and Dissemination, University of York. Cholesterol and coronary heart disease: screening and treatment. *Eff Health Care* 1998; **4**:1-16.

57. Burr ML, Fehily AM, Gilbert JF, *et al.* Effects of changes in fat, fish, and fibre intakes on death and myocardial reinfarction: diet and reinfarction trial (DART). *Lancet* 1989; **2**:757-61.

58. Appel LJ, Moore TJ, Obarzanek E, *et al.* A clinical trial of the effects of dietary patterns on blood pressure. *N Engl J Med* 1997; **336**:1117-24.

59. De Lorgeril M, Renaud S, Mamelle N, *et al.* Mediterranean alpha-linolenic acid-rich diet in secondary prevention of coronary heart disease [published erratum appears in *Lancet* 1995; **345**:738]. *Lancet* 1994; **343**:1454-9.

60. Graudal NA, Galloe AM, Garred P. Effects of sodium restriction on blood pressure, renin, aldosterone, catecholamines, cholesterols, and triglyceride: a meta-analysis. *JAMA* 1998; **279**:1383-91.

61. Whelton PK, Appel LJ, Espeland MA, *et al.* Sodium reduction and weight loss in the treatment of hypertension in older people: a randomized controlled trial of nonpharmacologic interventions in the elderly (TONE). TONE Collaborative Research Group [published erratum appears in *JAMA* 1998; **279**:1954]. *JAMA* 1998; **279**:839-46.

62. Midgley JP, Matthew AG, Greenwood CM, Logan AG. Effect of reduced dietary sodium on blood pressure: a meta-analysis of randomized controlled trials. *JAMA* 1996; **275**:1590-7.

63. Alderman MH, Madhavan S, Cohen H, Sealey JE, Laragh JH. Low urinary sodium is associated with greater risk of myocardial infarction among treated hypertensive men. *Hypertension* 1995; **25**:1144-52.

64. Brand MB, Mulrow CD, Chiquette E. Weight-reducing diets for control of hypertension in adults. (Cochrane Review) In: *The Cochrane Library*, Issue 4, 1998. Oxford: Update Software.

65. Hayden M, Pignone M, Phillips C, Mulrow C. *Aspirin chemoprophylaxis for the primary prevention of cardiovascular events: a systematic review for the U.S. Preventive Task Force*, Sep 2000. Agency for Healthcare Research and Quality contract no: 290-97-0011; project number: 6919-00003.

66. Hansson L, Zanchetti A, Carruthers SG, *et al.* Effects of intensive blood-pressure lowering and low-dose aspirin in patients with hypertension: principal results of the Hypertension Optimal Treatment (HOT) randomised trial. HOT Study Group. *Lancet* 1998; **351**:1755-62.

67. Steering Committee of the Physicians' Health Study Research Group. Final report on the aspirin component of the ongoing Physicians' Health Study. *N Engl J Med* 1989; **321**:129-35.

68. Meade TW, Brennan PJ. Determination of who may derive most benefit from aspirin in primary prevention: subgroup results from a randomised controlled trial. *BMJ* 2000; **321**:13-17.

69. The Women's Health Initiative Study Group. Design of the Women's Health Initiative clinical trial and observational study. *Control Clin Trials* 1998; **19**:61-109.

70. Antiplatelet Trialists' Collaboration. Collaborative overview of randomised trials of antiplatelet therapy – I: Prevention of death, myocardial infarction, and stroke by prolonged antiplatelet therapy in various categories of patients [published erratum appears in *BMJ* 1994; **308**:1540]. *BMJ* 1994; **308**:81-106.

71. CAPRIE Steering Committee. A randomised, blinded, trial of clopidogrel versus aspirin in patients at risk of ischaemic events (CAPRIE). *Lancet* 1996; **348**:1329-39.

72. Roderick PJ, Wilkes HC, Meade TW. The gastrointestinal toxicity of aspirin: an overview of randomised controlled trials. *Br J Clin Pharmacol* 1993; **35**:219-26.

73. Stalnikowicz-Darvasi R. Gastrointestinal bleeding during low-dose aspirin administration for prevention of arterial occlusive events. A critical analysis. *J Clin Gastroenterol* 1995; **21**:13-16.

74. Dickinson JP, Prentice CR. Aspirin: benefit and risk in thromboprophylaxis. *QJM* 1998; **91**:523-38.

75. Cappelleri JC, Lau J, Kupelnick B, Chalmers TC. Efficacy and safety of different aspirin dosages on vascular diseases in high-risk patients. A metaregression analysis [serial online]. *Online J Curr Clin Trials* 1995; Doc no 174.

76. Weil J, Colin-Jones D, Langman M, *et al.* Prophylactic aspirin and risk of peptic ulcer bleeding. *BMJ* 1995; **310**:827-30.

77. Kelly JP, Kaufman DW, Jurgelon JM, Sheehan J, Koff RS, Shapiro S. Risk of aspirin-associated major upper-gastrointestinal bleeding with enteric-coated or buffered product. *Lancet* 1996; **348**:1413-16.

78. Thun MJ, Peto R, Lopez AD, *et al*. Alcohol consumption and mortality among middle-aged and elderly U.S. adults. *N Engl J Med* 1997; **337**:1705-14.

79. Boffetta P, Garfinkel L. Alcohol drinking and mortality among men enrolled in an American Cancer Society prospective study. *Epidemiology* 1990; **1**:342-8.

80. Beilin LJ, Puddey IB, Burke V. Alcohol and hypertension—kill or cure? *J Hum Hypertens* 1996; **10**:S1-5.

81. Campbell NR, Ashley MJ, Carruthers SG, Lacourciere Y, McKay DW. Lifestyle modifications to prevent and control hypertension. 3. Recommendations on alcohol consumption. Canadian Hypertension Society, Canadian Coalition for High Blood Pressure Prevention and Control, Laboratory Centre for Disease Control at Health Canada, Heart and Stroke Foundation of Canada. *CMAJ* 1999; **160**:S13-20.

82. The Medical Research Council's General Practice Research Framework. Thrombosis prevention trial: randomised trial of low-intensity oral anticoagulation with warfarin and low-dose aspirin in the primary prevention of ischaemic heart disease in men at increased risk. *Lancet* 1998; **351**:233-41.

83. Anand SS, Yusuf S. Oral anticoagulant therapy in patients with coronary artery disease: a meta-analysis. *JAMA* 1999; **282**:2058-67.

84. Houtman JP. Trace elements and cardiovascular diseases. *J Cardiovasc Risk* 1996; **3**:18-25.

85. Neve J. Selenium as a risk factor for cardiovascular diseases. *J Cardiovasc Risk* 1996; **3**:42-7.

86. Lonn EM, Yusuf S. Is there a role for antioxidant vitamins in the prevention of cardiovascular diseases? An update on epidemiological and clinical trials data. *Can J Cardiol* 1997; **13**:957-65.

87. Jha P, Flather M, Lonn E, Farkouh M, Yusuf S. The antioxidant vitamins and cardiovascular disease. A critical review of epidemiologic and clinical trial data. *Ann Intern Med* 1995; **123**:860-72.

88. Rexrode KM, Manson JE. Antioxidants and coronary heart disease: observational studies. *J Cardiovasc Risk* 1996; **3**:363-7.

89. Gaziano JM. Randomized trials of dietary antioxidants in cardiovascular disease prevention and treatment. *J Cardiovasc Risk* 1996; **3**:368-71.

90. Egger M, Schneider M, Davey Smith G. Spurious precision? Meta-analysis of observational studies. *BMJ* 1998; **316**:140-4.

91. Rapola JM, Virtamo J, Ripatti S, *et al*. Randomised trial of alpha-tocopherol and beta-carotene supplements on incidence of major coronary events in men with previous myocardial infraction. *Lancet* 1997; **349**:1715-20.

92. Klipstein-Grobusch K, Geleijnse JM, Den Breeijen JH, *et al*. Dietary antioxidants and risk of myocardial infarction in the elderly: the Rotterdam Study. *Am J Clin Nutr* 1999; **69**:261-6.

93. Losonczy KG, Harris TB, Havlik RJ. Vitamin E and vitamin C supplement use and risk of all-cause and coronary heart disease mortality in older people: the Established Populations for Epidemiologic Studies of the Elderly. *Am J Clin Nutr* 1996; **64**:190-6.

94. Todd S, Woodward M, Tunstall-Pedoe H, Bolton-Smith C. Dietary antioxidant vitamins and fiber in the etiology of cardiovascular disease and all-causes mortality: results from the Scottish Heart Health Study. *Am J Epidemiol* 1999; **150**:1073-80.

95. Sahyoun NR, Jacques PF, Russell RM. Carotenoids, vitamins C and E, and mortality in an elderly population. *Am J Epidemiol* 1996; **144**:501-11.

96. Gruppo Italiano per lo Studio della Sopravvivenza nell'Infarto miocardico. Dietary supplementation with n-3 polyunsaturated fatty acids and vitamin E after myocardial infarction: results of the GISSI-Prevenzione trial. *Lancet* 1999; **354**:447-55.

97. Stephens NG, Parsons A, Schofield PM, Kelly F, Cheeseman K, Mitchinson MJ. Randomised controlled trial of vitamin E in patients with coronary disease: Cambridge Heart Antioxidant Study (CHAOS). *Lancet* 1996; **347**:781-6.

98. Yusuf S, Dagenais G, Pogue J, Bosch J, Sleight P. Vitamin E supplementation and cardiovascular events in high-risk patients. The Heart Outcomes Prevention Evaluation Study Investigators. *N Engl J Med* 2000; **342**:154-60.

99. Li JY, Taylor PR, Li B, *et al.* Nutrition intervention trials in Linxian, China: multiple vitamin/mineral supplementation, cancer incidence, and disease-specific mortality among adults with esophageal dysplasia. *J Natl Cancer Inst* 1993; **85**:1492-8.

100. Mark SD, Wang W, Fraumeni JF Jr, *et al.* Lowered risks of hypertension and cerebrovascular disease after vitamin/mineral supplementation: the Linxian Nutrition Intervention Trial. *Am J Epidemiol* 1996; **143**:658-64.

101. Morris MC, Sacks F, Rosner B. Does fish oil lower blood pressure? A meta-analysis of controlled trials. *Circulation* 1993; **88**:523-33.

102. Hertog MG, Feskens EJ, Hollman PC, Katan MB, Kromhout D. Dietary antioxidant flavonoids and risk of coronary heart disease: the Zutphen Elderly Study. *Lancet* 1993; **342**:1007-11.

103. Knekt P, Jarvinen R, Reunanen A, Maatela J. Flavonoid intake and coronary mortality in Finland: a cohort study. *BMJ* 1996; **312**:478-81.

104. Rimm EB, Katan MB, Ascherio A, Stampfer MJ, Willett WC. Relation between intake of flavonoids and risk for coronary heart disease in male health professionals. *Ann Intern Med* 1996; **125**:384-9.

105. Kromhout D. Diet-heart issues in a pharmacological era. *Lancet* 1996; **348**:S20-2.

106. Yochum L, Kushi LH, Meyer K, Folsom AR. Dietary flavonoid intake and risk of cardiovascular disease in postmenopausal women [published erratum appears in *Am J Epidemiol* 1999; **150**:432]. *Am J Epidemiol* 1999; **149**:943-9.

107. Ackerman RT, Mulrow CD, Ramirez G, Gardner CD, Morbidoni L, Lawrence VA. Garlic shows promise for improving some cardiovascular risk factors [in press]. *Arch Intern Med* 2000.

108. Whelton PK, He J, Cutler JA, *et al.* Effects of oral potassium on blood pressure. Meta-analysis of randomized controlled clinical trials. *JAMA* 1997; **277**:1624-32.

109. Griffith LE, Guyatt GH, Cook RJ, Bucher HC, Cook DJ. The influence of dietary and nondietary calcium supplementation on blood pressure: an updated metaanalysis of randomized controlled trials. *Am J Hypertens* 1999; **12**:84-92.

CHAPTER 5

How do we best individualize treatment for patients based on their cardiovascular risk profile?

Michael Pignone
Cynthia D Mulrow

What parameters should we consider when we help patients with multiple cardiovascular risk factors prioritize their treatments?

Which therapies will most benefit patients with hypertension and other cardiovascular risk factors, but no known cardiovascular disease?

Which therapies will most benefit patients with hypertension, other cardiovascular risk factors, and known cardiovascular disease?

How do we help prioritize and sequence various treatments for hypertensive patients with multiple cardiovascular risk factors?

Summary bottom lines

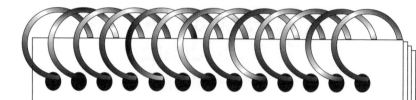

Patient Notes

Mr William Jones

- Retired city planner
- Hypertension
- 5-year CVD risk: 5%

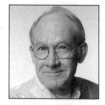

Mrs Elizabeth Jefferies

- Violinist
- Hypertension, diabetes, osteoarthritis
- 5-year CVD risk: 7%

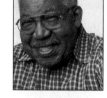

Mrs Pauline Smith

- School volunteer
- Hypertension, diabetes, dyslipidemia, sinusitis
- 5-year CVD risk: 10%

Mr Edward McIntosh

- Retired epidemiologist
- Hypertension, recent myocardial infarction
- 5-year CVD risk: 15%

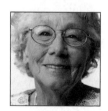

What parameters should we consider when we help patients with multiple cardiovascular risk factors prioritize their treatments?

In Chapter 3, we described tools that can be used to estimate cardiovascular prognosis for individual patients. In Chapter 4, we described treatments that are more likely to benefit than harm patients with hypertension. We described several effective therapies for hypertensive patients with and without known cardiovascular disease (see Tables 4.1 and 4.2, Chapter 4). In this chapter, we discuss methods for integrating and prioritizing therapies for individual patients with various cardiovascular risk profiles.

We believe assessment of individual risk is necessary to optimize decisions about who to treat with what therapy. Such assessment identifies important comorbid cardiovascular risk factors that may warrant treatment, and helps establish the amount of absolute benefit that patients can expect from particular therapies. We also believe that the benefits of treating hypertensive individuals vary, depending upon each person's competing risks of dying from noncardiovascular-related causes. For example, a patient with multiple serious conditions, such as end-stage Alzheimer's disease, obstructive lung disease, frequent falls, gout, and urinary incontinence, has high competing risks that may minimize or negate the benefits of treating hypertension.

We find prioritization of treatments for patients with multiple cardiovascular risk factors and multiple conditions very difficult. Multiple parameters, such as those given in Box 5.1, deserve consideration. Knowing and weighing the parameters across multiple risk factors, conditions, and therapies is laudable, but often not achievable. Explaining them to patients is daunting and time-consuming. Some patients are more interested in our "bottom line, authoritative" recommendations than they are in obtaining diverse, complicated information necessary to make their own or joint informed decisions. Nevertheless, we advocate informed joint decision-making, with attention to the parameters given in Box 5.1, when possible.

> **Box 5.1. Parameters that help prioritize among various treatments for patients.**
>
> - Type and immediacy of expected benefits
> - Magnitude of expected benefits
> - Type and immediacy of expected harms
> - Magnitude of expected harms
> - Availability and costs of treatments
> - Feasibility, likely adherence with treatments
> - Competing risks from various conditions
> - Expected interactions with other treatments
> - Patient and provider preferences and values

 # Which therapies will most benefit patients with hypertension and other cardiovascular risk factors, but no known cardiovascular disease?

Types of benefits that can be expected from treatment of hypertension and other cardiovascular risk factors include fewer deaths and longer survival times, and less fatal and nonfatal cardiovascular disease, such as myocardial infarction and stroke. Table 5.1 shows the approximate magnitude of such benefits that can be expected from particular therapies in people without known cardiovascular disease. The magnitude of risk reduction for cardiovascular disease is similar for antihypertensive and lipid-lowering drug therapy; it is slightly lower for aspirin prophylaxis. Both the type and magnitude of benefits that can be expected from lifestyle interventions, such as exercising more or quitting smoking, are less clear.

Of note, some benefits occur immediately, such as those from aspirin, while others may require a year or more of treatment, such as those from lipid-lowering therapy. The effect of long-term treatment for more than ten years is unknown for all of the interventions. Finally, some of the interventions, such as quitting smoking, have multiple benefits including decreased risk of lung cancer and respiratory disease, that are not shown.

Table 5.1. Approximate relative risk reductions associated with various treatments for hypertensive people with other cardiovascular risk factors but no known cardiovascular disease

Therapy	Approximate relative risk reduction for death (range)	Approximate relative risk reduction for cardiovascular disease (range)
ACE inhibitor (ramipril)	15% (5% to 25%)	20% (15% to 30%)
Antiglycemic drug therapy	Not demonstrated	Not demonstrated
Antihypertensive drug therapy	10% (5% to 20%)	30% (15% to 40%)
Antilipidemic drug therapy	5% (20% reduction to 10% increase)	30% (20% to 40%)
Aspirin	5% (15% reduction to 5% increase)	15% (5% to 30%)
Physical activity	Unclear	Unclear
Smoking cessation	Unclear, as much as 20% or more	Unclear, as much as 50%

Which therapies will most benefit patients with hypertension, other cardiovascular risk factors, and known cardiovascular disease?

Patients with hypertension and known cardiovascular disease are at high risk of future cardiovascular events and warrant aggressive risk factor management. We found that several different effective therapeutic options, given in Table 4.2, are available. We found little data that addressed how the different therapies interacted with one another to reduce risk. As more marked degrees of abnormalities of risk factors are associated with higher risks, we usually prioritize treatment of extremely abnormal levels of blood pressure or lipids over treatment of mildly abnormal levels of these or other risk factors. Table 5.2 shows approximate risk reductions that can be expected with different treatments for patients with known cardiovascular disease.

Table 5.2. Approximate relative risk reductions associated with various treatments for hypertensive people with other cardiovascular risk factors and known cardiovascular disease

Therapy	Approximate relative risk reduction for death (range)	Approximate relative risk reduction for cardiovascular disease (range)
ACE inhibitor (ramipril)	15% (5% to 25%)	20% (15% to 30%)
Antiglycemic drug therapy	Not demonstrated	Not demonstrated
Antilipidemic drug therapy[a]	20% (10% to 30%)	30% (20% to 40%)
Aspirin	15% (10% to 20%)	25% (10% to 40%)
Beta-blockers	25% (15% to 30%)	25% (10% to 40%)
Cardiac rehabilitation	25% (10% to 40%)	25% (10% to 40%)
Fish oil	15% (5% to 25%)	10% (0% to 20%)
Mediterranean diet	30% (10% to 80%)	30% (45% to 85%)
Smoking cessation	Unclear, as much as 20% or more	Unclear, as much as 50%

[a] Applies primarily to statin treatment for elevations in LDL and total cholesterol. Treatment with fibrates for near normal LDL and total cholesterol, but low levels of HDL cholesterol, has shown risk reductions of approximately 10% for death and 25% for cardiovascular disease.

How do we help prioritize and sequence various treatments for hypertensive patients with multiple cardiovascular risk factors?

We have no profound illuminations regarding fail-safe methods for helping patients prioritize treatment preferences. We believe that decisions about which therapies should be used together and the order in which they should be initiated depends upon the following:

- The types of benefits that patients are most interested in
- The patient's individual risk profile and comorbid conditions
- The degree of modifiability of risk and comorbid conditions
- The effect size of available treatments
- The types and frequency of harms found with particular treatments
- The availability, complexity, feasibility, and costs of particular therapies
- Whether patients think they are ready to adhere to particular therapies
- The degree of certainty or uncertainty of assessments

When facing patients with multiple risk factors and conditions, we ideally use the above principles to guide our discussions regarding which therapies should be tried and when. When possible, we use balance sheets and decision aids, such as Table 4.4 addressing benefits and harms of aspirin in Chapter 4 and the sample shown in Box 5.2, to guide discussions. As available data suggest that the relative risk reductions that can be achieved with particular therapies are generally independent of underlying cardiovascular risk levels, we project absolute benefits of treatments for individual patients based on their own individual risk profiles. Thus, patients at higher risk stand to gain more from treatment over the next five to ten years than patients at lower risk, and are less likely to have the benefits of treatment offset by other harms. Ideally, we try to reach agreement with patients about what constitutes sufficient enough risk to warrant starting and/or adding treatment.

Box 5.2. Decision tool for patients without known cardiovascular disease.

Name	Mr Singh	
Age	85	years
Systolic blood pressure	160	mm Hg
Total cholesterol	20	mg/dl
HDL cholesterol	38	mg/dl

Sex	●	Male	○	Female
Smoker	○	Yes	●	No
Diabetes	○	Yes	●	No
ECG-based LVH	●	Yes	○	No
Risk Time Range	5	Years		

Mr Singh, your risk of having a cardiovascular event, such as a stroke or heart attack, in the next five years is about 25%. By comparison, an 85-year-old man with no risk factors has about a 15% chance of having such events in the next five years.

The graph shows your risk.

5-year risk for cardiovascular events

Low ◆ High

0%　5%　10%　15%　20%　25%　30%

A number of treatments are available to you that may help prevent future cardiovascular problems. Some are listed below:

☐ Aspirin
☑ Blood pressure medication
☐ Lipid medication

Select an intervention
⬅

Box 5.2 continued. Decision tool for patients without known cardiovascular disease.

Taking medication to lower your blood pressure reduces your chance of having a heart attack or stroke, and several medications are available for this purpose. On average, these medications lower the chance of having a heart attack or stroke by about 30%. The graph below shows your own chance of having a heart attack or stroke would be decreased from about 25% to about 15%. They also reduce the chance of developing heart failure — a condition in which your heart does not pump the blood well, causing swelling in the legs and shortness of breath — by 50%.

Several different medications are available for treating hypertension. Your choice of medications will depend on many factors, including the cost and side effects of the medications and the presence of other illnesses that may be helped or worsened by the medication used to treat high blood pressure.

Risk of heart attack or stroke after adding blood pressure medication

Low								High
0%	5%	10%	15%	20%	25%	30%	

Adapted from tool developed by Michael Pignone, MD, MPH: www.med-decisions.com/cvtool

---

To help prioritize for patients without known cardiovascular disease, we try to estimate the amount of risk associated with each of the patient's risk factors and conditions, using tools such as those described in Chapter 3. We tie our estimate of benefit from a particular therapy to our estimate of risk from a particular factor or condition. For example, we postulate that a patient with especially abnormal levels of a risk factor, such as severe hypertension, may benefit more from having his or her hypertension treated than by taking an aspirin.

We do inform patients about the types of benefits and harms that they might expect from particular treatments. For example, primary prevention trials show that aspirin and lipid lowering statin drugs both reduce risk of coronary heart disease, but probably not stroke. Aspirin is much less expensive than statin drugs, but it precipitates more adverse effects, such as gastrointestinal bleeding. Some patients' choices between using an aspirin or a statin or both may depend on the costs of the drugs and their perceived risks of adverse effects. Other patients' choices may be more dependent upon their perceived benefits of treatments. For example, some patients may prefer to stop smoking rather than taking either an aspirin or a statin, because of perceived multiple benefits of smoking cessation, and fewer perceived benefits from the aspirin or statin. Other patients may feel that they are not ready or able to quit smoking, yet they are ready and able to take medications.

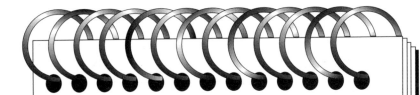

Patient Notes

Mr William Jones

- Hypertension
- 5-year CVD risk: 5%

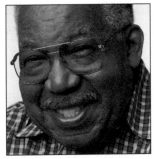

Clinician's actions

- Advised that antihypertensive therapy with a low-dose diuretic or ACE inhibitor would reduce Mr. Jones' five-year chance (relative risk) of death by about 10% and reduce his chance (relative risk) of a CVD event by about 30%. Advised that such treatment would decrease Mr Jones' five-year probability of having a CVD event from about 5% to about 3% (absolute risk). Advised of potential side effects of diuretics and ACE inhibitors.
- Advised that aspirin prophylaxis would reduce his five-year chance of a CVD event by about 15%, would not affect his risk of death, and would increase his risk of major gastrointestinal bleeding by 0.1–0.2% per year.

Mr Jones' informed decision

- Chooses antihypertensive therapy with a low-dose diuretic.

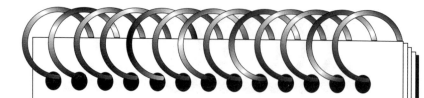

Patient Notes

Mrs Elizabeth Jefferies

- Hypertension, diabetes, arthritis
- 5-year CVD risk: 7%

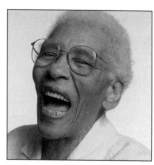

Clinician's action

- Advised that antihypertensive therapy with an ACE inhibitor would reduce Mrs Jefferies' chance of CVD events by 20%, from an absolute risk of 7% over 5 years to about 5.5% over 5 years. Advised that adding aspirin would reduce her chance of CVD events by 15%, from 5.5% to 4.5% over 5 years, and would increase her risk of major GI bleeding by more than 0.1- 0.2% per year. Advised that her current NSAIDs that she takes for arthritis might interfere with her antihypertensive therapy and increase her blood pressure (see Chapter 7), and that stopping her NSAIDs would decrease her bleeding risks. Advised that the benefits of antiglycemic therapy are unclear but that her chances of retinopathy and albuminuria would be decreased.

Mrs Jefferies' informed decision

- Chooses aspirin, ACE inhibitor, and antiglycemic therapy. Chooses to continue her NSAIDs as well as the aspirin despite increased bleeding risks because she wants to be pain free and other pain therapies have not worked for her in the past.

Patient Notes

Mrs Pauline Smith

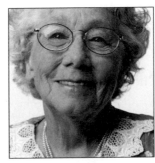

- Hypertension, diabetes, dyslipidemia, sinusitis
- 5-year CVD risk: 10%

Clinician's action

- Advised that aspirin would reduce Mrs Smith's relative risk of CVD by 15%, an ACE inhibitor by 20%, and a lipid lowering agent by 30%. Advised that taking a lipid lowering drug would reduce her absolute risk from 10% to 7% over 5 years. Adding an ACE inhibitor would likely reduce her absolute risk further to about 5.5% over 5 years, and adding an aspirin would reduce her absolute risk to 4.5% over 5 years. The aspirin would also increase her risk of a major gastrointestinal bleed by 0.1–0.2%. Advised that aspirin is less expensive than the lipid lowering drug and the ACE inhibitor, and that all involve taking single daily doses.

Mrs Smith's informed decision

- Chooses to use the statin drug and ACE inhibitor, but not to take aspirin as the increase in risk of bleeding was too close to the additional benefit of reducing a cardiovascular event. She says all of this information about her hypertension, diabetes, and cholesterol is well and good, but what are we going to do about the sinusitis that is bothering her now?

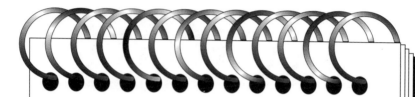

Patient Notes

Mr Edward McIntosh

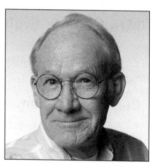

- Hypertension, recent myocardial infarction
- 5-year CVD risk: 15%

Clinician's action

- Advised that switching from a current high-fat, fast-food diet to a Mediterranean-type diet could reduce Mr McIntosh's relative risk of death and future myocardial infarctions by about 30% to 50% in the next two to five years. Advised that this means an absolute risk reduction for him from his current five-year risk of 15% to around 7% or 10%. Advised that aspirin, a beta-blocker, and cardiac rehabilitation could each reduce his relative risks of CVD by about 25%, or from 15% to 11%. Advised that combining effective interventions such as beta-blockers and aspirin will likely reduce risks further than either intervention alone. Advised that fish oil supplements alone could reduce relative risk of recurrent myocardial infarction by about 10%, but that added benefits of fish oil supplements over consuming Mediterranean-type diets are unclear. Advised regarding potential adverse effects of therapies and their costs.

Mr McIntosh's informed decision

- Chooses to initiate therapy with a beta-blocker and adopt a Mediterranean diet. He decides against aspirin therapy because of a history of stomach upset when he has used aspirin in the past. Unfortunately, he opts out of cardiac rehabilitation, claiming lack of time and inconvenience.

Summary bottom lines

- Use the following parameters to help patients with multiple risk factors and conditions prioritize their treatments (Consensus opinion):
  - Assess the types of benefits that patients are most interested in.
  - Assess the patient's individual risk profile and comorbid conditions.
  - Estimate the degree of modifiability of risk and comorbid conditions.
  - Consider the effect size of available treatments.
  - Review the types and frequency of harms found with particular treatments.
  - Review the availability, complexity, feasibility, and costs of particular therapies.
  - Ask whether patients think they are ready to adhere to particular therapies.
  - Be honest about your degree of certainty or uncertainty of assessments.
- Do not forget to address patient's other comorbid conditions, and to stay within the time constraints of busy clinic schedules! (Consensus opinion)
- When available, use written materials and decision aids to help guide discussions. (Consensus opinion)

CHAPTER 6

How do we individualize antihypertensive therapy for patients with specific comorbid conditions?

Michael Pignone
Stacey Sheridan
Cynthia D Mulrow

When should the presence of comorbid conditions affect initial choices of antihypertensive drugs?

*Which comorbid conditions **have good indications to prescribe** specific antihypertensive therapies?*

*Which comorbid conditions **do not have good indications to prescribe** specific antihypertensive therapies?*

*Which comorbid conditions **have good indications to avoid** specific antihypertensive therapies?*

*Which comorbid conditions **do not have good indications to avoid** specific antihypertensive therapies?*

*Which comorbid conditions **have significant clinical trade-offs** in prescribing or avoiding specific antihypertensive therapies?*

*Which comorbid conditions **have insufficient evidence to either prescribe or avoid** specific antihypertensive therapies?*

Summary bottom lines

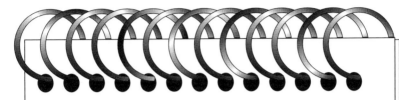

Patient Notes

Mr William Lee, age 55, corporate sales executive

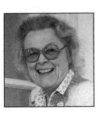

- Takes HCTZ for hypertension

Reason for visit

- Three gouty attacks in the last 12 months

Clinical findings

- BP 142/86 mm Hg

Clinical question

Should possible drug-related adverse effects influence our choice of antihypertensive therapy in adults with specific comorbid conditions such as gout?

Mrs Marjorie Poindexter, age 74, retired

- Takes HCTZ for hypertension

Reason for visit

- Follow-up of hypertension and frequent migraines

Clinical findings

- BP 165/90 mm Hg

Clinical question

When should a comorbid condition, such as migraine headaches, influence our choice of antihypertensive agents?

When should the presence of comorbid conditions affect initial choices of antihypertensive drugs?

In the following sections we examine several health conditions that may affect the choice of initial antihypertensive therapy. These conditions fall into two categories: (1) conditions in which a particular therapy may offer particular specific benefits, and (2) conditions for which certain therapies may cause particular harms.

Which comorbid conditions have good indications to prescribe specific antihypertensive therapies?

Coronary artery disease

Angina

We found a meta-analysis of multiple randomized trials that compared antianginal drugs such as beta-blockers and calcium channel blockers. Rates of myocardial infarction or cardiac death were similar between groups.[1](Tx:LIa) Overall, beta-blockers were slightly more successful than calcium channel blockers in reducing anginal episodes (0.31 fewer episodes per week; 95% CI 0.00 to 0.62). Also, there were fewer withdrawals from adverse effects with beta-blockers compared with calcium channel blockers. However, when calcium channel blockers other than nifedipine were compared with beta-blockers, there was no difference in anginal events or withdrawal rates. Longer-acting calcium channel blockers appeared to perform moderately better than short-acting agents, but the differences were not statistically significant.

Our practiced judgments

In patients with angina and hypertension, we prefer beta-blockers for initial therapy if there are no strong contraindications, such as severe asthma. We use long-acting calcium channel blockers, other than nifedipine, when beta-blockers cannot be used or when additional agents are needed for control of symptoms. We also consider ACE inhibitors concomitantly for high-risk patients with angina and hypertension. ACE inhibitors may decrease myocardial infarctions and improve survival, although their effect on angina symptoms is unclear (see below).

Myocardial infarction

We found several randomized controlled trials that showed patients who have had a myocardial infarction with no evidence of systolic dysfunction live longer when they are given long-term beta-blocker therapy.[2](Tx:LIa) Pooled analyses show that the odds of death are reduced by 23% (odds ratio 0.77; 95% CI 0.69 to 0.85) in patients receiving long-term beta-blocker therapy compared with those receiving placebo. The risk of nonfatal reinfarction was reduced by 24% (95% CI 11% to 36%). Of note, beta-blockers with intrinsic sympathomimetic acitivity should not be used.

We found one large trial in patients at high-risk of cardiovascular disease that showed an ACE inhibitor, ramipril, reduced the risk of death by 16% and the risk of cardiovascular events by 22% (relative risk 0.78; 95% CI 0.70 to 0.86) compared with placebo.[3](Tx:LIb) In this trial, approximately 52% of the participants had previously had a myocardial infarction, 47% had hypertension, and 40% were taking beta-blockers. We found multiple trials that showed various ACE inhibitors reduced cardiovascular morbidity and/or mortality after myocardial infarction in patients with left ventricular systolic dysfunction.[4](Tx:LIa)

Please see the section that describes conditions with indications to avoid specific drugs for discussion of calcium channel blockers in people with myocardial infarction.

Our practiced judgments

We routinely prescribe beta-blockers without intrinsic sympathomimetic activity for patients with hypertension and myocardial infarction. We routinely concomitantly prescribe ACE inhibitors for patients with hypertension and myocardial infarction complicated by left ventricular systolic dysfunction. In patients with known left ventricular systolic dysfunction, we titrate beta-blocker doses very slowly and avoid them if patients have acute exacerbations of heart failure symptoms. We routinely avoid calcium channel blockers, such as diltiazem, in patients with hypertension, recent myocardial infarction, and left ventricular systolic dysfunction. In patients with hypertension, myocardial infarction, left ventricular systolic dysfunction, and symptomatic angina despite ACE inhibitors, beta-blockers, and nitrates, we consider adding amlodipine and/or revascularization.

Diabetes

We found multiple randomized trials that showed antihypertensive therapy reduced cardiovascular disease morbidity and mortality in people with diabetes.[5](Tx:LIa) ACE inhibitors, beta-blockers, and low dose thiazide diuretics were proven effective agents, and one large trial reported no difference in renal disease between diabetic patients randomized to a beta-blocker or ACE inhibitor.[6](Tx:L1b) We found two trials that reported hypertensive diabetic patients who were randomized to take an ACE inhibitor had fewer coronary heart disease events than patients randomized to a calcium channel blocker (nisoldipine or amlodipine).[7,8](Tx:L1b)

We found a cohort study of over 12000 American adults aged 45 to 64 that reported patients with hypertension who were taking thiazide diuretics, calcium channel blockers, or ACE inhibitors had no difference in the rate of developing diabetes than patients on no therapy.[9](H:L2b) Patients taking beta-blockers had a relative hazard for diabetes of 1.28 (95% CI 1.04 to 1.57) after adjustment for potential confounders.

We also found a large trial that showed fewer cardiovascular events in diabetics who had more tightly controlled blood pressure levels (below 150/85 mm Hg) compared to less tightly controlled blood pressures (below 180/105 mm Hg).[10] (Please see Chapter 7 for more information regarding blood pressure targets in people with and without diabetes. Of note, antiglycemic therapy for Type 2 diabetes may decrease retinopathy albuminuria but has no significant demonstrated effects on myocardial infarction or stroke.)

Our practiced judgments

We consider ACE inhibitors, beta-blockers, or low dose thiazide diuretics appropriate choices for patients with Type 2 diabetes. However, we generally advise our diabetic patients with either Type 1 or Type 2 diabetes to take an ACE inhibitor. In patients with Type 1 or 2 diabetes and previous myocardial infarction, we routinely advise use of both ACE inhibitors and beta-blockers.

Heart failure from left ventricular systolic dysfunction

ACE inhibitors and heart failure

We found a systematic review of multiple placebo controlled trials that showed ACE inhibitors added to diuretic therapy decreased rates of hospitalizations, recurrent myocardial infarctions, and death (summary odds ratio for death 0.65; 95% CI 0.57 to 0.74) in patients with heart failure due to systolic dysfunction.[4](Tx:L1a) The largest benefits were found in patients who had ejection fractions less than 25% and occurred within the first 90 days of initiating therapy. We found effects were similar across New York Heart Association classes (NYHA) I through IV and in patients with ischemic and nonischemic heart failure. The percentage of patients with both heart failure and hypertension was not reported in the systematic review, but as many as one-third to one-half of the patients in some of the trials had known hypertension.

Angiotensin II receptor blockers and heart failure

Although angiotensin II receptor blockers improve outcomes in people with left ventricular failure, we found no large randomized trials that demonstrate their effects on morbidity or mortality in people with hypertension.

Beta-blockers and heart failure

We found several systematic reviews and meta-analyses that examined the effect of beta-blockers on patients with heart failure from systolic dysfunction.[1,11-13](Tx:L1a) Trials consistently showed reductions in total mortality of 30% among patients assigned to standard therapy plus beta-blockers compared with standard therapy and placebo. Standard therapy typically includes ACE inhibitors, thiazide or loop diuretics, and possibly digoxin and/or Aldactone. The percentage of patients with both heart failure and hypertension generally was not reported in the systematic reviews.

Calcium channel blockers and heart failure

We found a review of three randomized trials that have evaluated whether different calcium channel blockers improve or worsen clinical outcomes in people with left ventricular systolic dysfunction;[14](Tx:L2b) findings have been mixed. One of the trials in patients already treated with diuretics and ACE inhibitors found no differences in combined survival and hospitalization rates between amlodipine and placebo (relative risk reduction 8%; 95% CI –6% to 21%).[15](Tx:L2b) Subgroup analysis from this trial suggested that patients with primary cardiomyopathy may have improved survival with amlodipine compared to placebo (relative risk reduction 25%; 95% CI 0.2% to 45%). A second small trial in people with idiopathic dilated cardiomyopathy found no survival differences with diltiazem compared to placebo but increased exercise tolerance and perceived quality of life with diltiazem.[14](Tx:L2b) A third trial found no differences in clinical outcomes between felodipine and placebo in patients with NYHA class ll to lll heart failure.[14](Tx:L2b) Large trials are continuing to evaluate whether benefits of specific calcium channel blockers outweigh their risks.

Our practiced judgments

We advise all patients with heart failure due to left ventricular systolic dysfunction to take ACE inhibitors unless they are contraindicated. We also advise patients with stable heart failure symptoms and left ventricular systolic dysfunction to take beta-blockers. We avoid calcium channel blockers other than amlodipine and short-acting alpha-blockers in patients with left ventricular systolic dysfunction. (For information on alpha-blockers, see the section that describes conditions that have good indications to avoid specific drugs.)

Migraine headaches

Migraine is a common disorder affecting about 6% of men and 15% to 18% of women, predominantly between the ages of 25 and 55 years of age.[16] While most migraneurs require only symptomatic treatment, some are placed on prophylactic migraine therapy due to multiple or severe attacks. To the extent that this population overlaps with the population requiring long-term antihypertensive therapy, it makes sense to choose an agent effective for both hypertension therapy and migraine prophylaxis.

We found several agents that have been used to treat hypertension also have been used to prevent migraine. These agents fall broadly into three categories: beta-blockers, calcium channel blockers, and central alpha-blockers. Of these classes, beta-blockers have been the most tested and the most preferred among neurologists and primary care physicians.[17] Wide variation in the efficacy of the drugs in this class and the drugs in the other two classes, however, mandates a close look at individual agents.

Unfortunately, many studies about individual agents have reached conflicting conclusions, reflecting differences in study design and scientific rigor. In several cases, the studies with the largest numbers of subjects have been of poorer methodological quality than the smaller studies. Formal meta-analysis has been difficult because of variable definitions, methods, and outcomes in the studies. One of the more recent and rigorous attempts to appraise the available information on prophylactic migraine treatment involved the following: (1) collecting all randomized double-blind placebo controlled trials of migraine prophylaxis that appeared in the English language between 1966 and 1996; (2) assigning a scientific rigor score from 1 for minimal to 5 for excellent for each study; and (3) averaging the scientific scores and results of the studies for each drug.[17] This approach weighted small studies as much as larger studies and provided ranges of benefit instead of point estimates. Nonetheless, it provides a useful framework for our discussion.

Beta-blockers

The above mentioned review found 16 of 18 randomized double-blind, placebo-controlled trials that consistently demonstrated that propranolol is more effective than placebo in the prophylaxis of migraine with a benefit of reduced migraine frequency ranging from 10% to 74%.[17](Tx:LIa) Similar results were found in a second meta-analysis of 28 controlled and open label trials.[18](Tx:LIa) There was no difference in efficacy among patients with classic versus common migraine, nor among patients who received different doses of propranolol. Less improvement was noted among people with a longer duration of chronic headaches and among people who recorded the treatment effects as part of a chronic daily diary rather than citing them from memory.

The review reported three well-designed trials that demonstrated a 28% to 33% reduction in migraine frequency among people taking 100 mg to 200 mg of metoprolol.[17](Tx:L1a) Additionally, one large randomized double-blind, placebo-controlled trial involving 200 migraneurs showed a 39% reduction in headache frequency with 5 mg of bisoprolol, one of the newer beta-1-selective adrenergic antagonists.[19](Tx:L1b) Results for atenolol and timolol have been mixed, with a few studies showing efficacy equivalent to propranolol and a few showing no significant benefit over placebo.[17](Tx:L2b) Trials of acebutolol, pindolol, oxprenolol, and alprenolol have been few, of poor scientific rigor, and without benefit over placebo.[17](Tx:L2b)

Calcium channel blockers

We found four small, randomized double-blind, placebo controlled trials of verapamil in patients with migraines.(Tx:L2b) Three showed verapamil compared to placebo decreased migraine frequency by 18% to 52%.[20-22] One showed a nonstatistically significant trend toward reducing migraine frequency that was consistent with those reported in the other studies.[23] Taken together, the trials suggested a dose-response relationship: migraine frequency decreased 15% with verapamil 240 mg daily and 50% with verapamil 320 mg daily.

Several small trials suggested flunarizine was associated with a 38% reduction in migraine frequency after four weeks of therapy.[17](Tx:L2b) Results of the prophylactic trials of nifedipine and nimodipine were mixed.

Central alpha antagonists

We found six randomized double-blind, placebo controlled trials that addressed whether clonidine decreased migraine frequency.[17](Tx:L2b) They had mixed results. Three studies suggested clonidine decreased migraine frequency by 10% to 29%, and three showed no benefit.

Our practiced judgments

We conclude beta-blockers, particularly propranolol and metoprolol, reduce migraine frequency. Because beta-blockers also have as good, or stronger, general evidence of effectiveness than calcium channel blockers for patients without special indications, we consider them the preferred agent in patients with hypertension and migraine. We do not preferentially advise clonidine in patients with migraine.

Nondiabetic renal disease

We found a meta-analysis of ten randomized trials that examined the effect of ACE inhibitors on nondiabetic renal disease.[24](Tx:L1a) Trials were conducted among patients with a variety of causes of renal failure and compared ACE inhibitors with other therapy such as beta-blockers, calcium channel blockers, or placebo. Most, but not all, of the studies examined patients with hypertension. Mean serum creatinine at baseline ranged from 1.0 to 4.4 mg/dL. The risk of progression to renal failure was lower for those taking ACE inhibitors compared to other agents or controls (relative risk 0.70; 95% CI 0.51 to 0.97). Reported risks of death with ACE inhibitors compared to controls were imprecise (relative risk 1.24; 95% CI 0.55 to 2.83).

We found an additional review that summarized trial data regarding effects of ACE inhibitor therapy on serum creatinine in patients with renal insufficiency.[25](Tx:L1a) Although many patients in the trials had acute worsening of glomerular filtration and serum creatinine when an ACE inhibitor was introduced, long-term progression of renal disease was less frequent among people given ACE inhibitors compared to controls.

Our practiced judgments

We routinely consider ACE inhibitors for patients with mild to moderate impaired renal function and hypertension.

Perioperative situations

We found two randomized trials that examined whether beta-blockers given perioperatively improved cardiovascular outcomes among 312 patients undergoing noncardiac surgery.[26, 27](Tx:L1b) Participants in both trials either had coronary artery disease or were considered high-risk for cardiovascular complications. In one trial, atenolol given intravenously immediately prior to surgery and orally after surgery for the length of the hospitalization significantly decreased two-year mortality compared with placebo (10% versus 21%, *p*=0.019).[26] In the second trial, bisoprolol given perioperatively, compared with placebo, significantly decreased death from coronary artery disease or nonfatal myocardial infarction within 30 days of surgery (3.5% versus 34%, *p*<0.001).[27]

Our practiced judgments

We recommend perioperative beta-blockers for patients with poorly controlled or previously untreated hypertension who are undergoing surgery and have no major contraindications such as severe asthma. We also add beta-blockers to current medications for patients with well-controlled hypertension and moderate to high cardiac risk who are undergoing surgery and have no contraindications.

Which comorbid conditions do not have good indications to prescribe specific antihypertensive therapies?

Lipid abnormalities

Lipid abnormalities are often present in patients with hypertension; both lipid abnormalities and hypertension contribute to increased risk of coronary heart disease and stroke. When selecting an antihypertensive agent, clinicians and patients must consider the evidence about the effect of the antihypertensive drug on lipid levels along with the evidence about the general effectiveness of the agent in preventing coronary heart disease and stroke events. A treatment may adversely affect lipid levels but still produce a net benefit on the risk of cardiovascular disease events. It also may improve lipid levels but fail to reduce or even increase cardiovascular disease events.

We found a meta-analysis of multiple controlled and uncontrolled trials that examined effects of different antihypertensive agents on lipid levels.[28](Tx:LIa) Table 6.1 summarizes pooled analyses of 474 of these trials that included more than 65 000 participants.

Table 6.1. Antihypertensive agents' effect on lipid levels (all units in mmol/L).

Drug class	Total cholesterol	Low-density lipoprotein	High-density lipoprotein	Triglycerides
Diuretics (low dose)	0.13 (0.09 to 0.18)	No change	No change	0.10 (0.03 to 0.18)
Beta-blocker (non-ISA)	No change	No change	−0.10 (−0.12 to −0.08)	0.35 (0.31 to 0.39)
Calcium antagonist	No change	No change	No change	No change
ACE inhibitor	No change	No change	No change	−0.07 (0.12 to −0.02)
Alpha-blocker	−0.23 (−0.28 to −0.18)	−0.20 (−0.25 to -0.15)	0.02 (0.01 to 0.04)	−0.07 (0.11 to −0.03)

The meta-analyses cited above suggested low-dose diuretics modestly increased total cholesterol (0.13 mmol/L or 5 mg/dL) and triglyceride levels and had no effects on LDL and HDL levels. Effects appeared greater in trials with large proportions of black participants. High-dose diuretics (data not shown) produced larger increases in total cholesterol (additional 0.12 mmol/L) and also increased LDL levels (0.19 mmol/L). Beta-blockers modestly increased triglycerides and decreased HDL cholesterol levels. Calcium antagonists and ACE inhibitors had little or no effect on lipid levels. Alpha-blockers decreased total cholesterol, LDL, and triglyceride levels, and increased HDL levels slightly. We found a randomized controlled trial published subsequent to the meta-analysis that showed, over two years, people receiving diuretics and lifestyle modification advice improved their lipid profiles (decrease of 0.12 mmol/L).[29](Tx:LIb)

We could not estimate the clinical consequences of observed changes in lipid levels with specific antihypertensive agents. We found agents, such as diuretics and beta-blockers, may have some negative effects on lipid levels, but they clearly decrease major morbid and mortal events in people with hypertension (Chapter 4).(Tx:LI) We found other agents such as the alpha-blocker, doxazosin, may have positive effects on lipid levels, but short-acting formulations increase the incidence of congestive heart failure and do not reduce ischemic events compared with chlorthalidone, a diuretic.[30](Tx:LIb)

Our practiced judgments

We conclude that the direct beneficial cardiovascular effects of specific antihypertensive agents, such as diuretics and beta-blockers, outweigh any changes in surrogate outcomes like lipid levels. We believe that the absolute clinical benefits of treating people with moderate to severe hypertension with low-dose diuretics and beta-blockers are likely much larger than any harmful effects mediated through lipid levels. We believe, in patients with mild hypertension, that harmful effects of specific antihypertensive agents on lipids could mitigate much of the direct beneficial effects on clinical outcomes. However, in the absence of strong data supporting this latter hypothesis, we do not choose agents other than low-dose diuretics or beta-blockers because of potential, yet unproven, adverse clinical effects.

Smoking

We found a meta-analysis of trials of clonidine for smoking cessation that includes six trials of 12 weeks duration.[31](Tx:LI) Three of the trials evaluated oral clonidine 0.15 to 0.45 mg daily and three evaluated transdermal clonidine patches 0.1 to 0.3 mg daily. Clonidine increased the odds of successful cessation (pooled odds ratio 1.89; 95% CI 1.30 to 2.74). These odds are similar to those found with nicotine replacement. The authors estimated that, on the average, this increase would translate to a 9% absolute increase in quit rate if the baseline quit rate was 14%.[31]

We found no long-term studies of the effect of clonidine on smoking cessation maintenance. Adverse effects, such as dry mouth and sedation, were common with clonidine, making it a poor choice for first-line smoking cessation therapy.

Our practiced judgments

We do not advise choosing clonidine as the agent of choice for hypertension in patients who also want to stop smoking. It is no more effective than other smoking cessation therapies, has important adverse effects, and has no proven morbidity or mortality benefits.

 # Which comorbid conditions have good indications to avoid specific antihypertensive therapies?

Obstructive airways disease: asthma and chronic obstructive pulmonary disease

Since their introduction, beta-blockers have been implicated in exacerbations of airway disease. Through the 1970s and 1980s much research categorized new beta-blockers according to the type of receptors they activated. Beta-1-receptor antagonists were mostly selective for the heart and the beta-2-receptor antagonists were mostly selective for the lungs and vasculature. Much work was done to evaluate which of these agents were effective and safe in which patients.

We found studies that reported airway exacerbation usually measured physiologic parameters such as airway resistance and forced expiratory volume in short-term, often single-dose, pre-post designs.(Tx:L2b) Treatment for underlying obstructive lung disease was discontinued just prior to testing, leading to confusion about whether the worsening parameters were secondary to discontinuance of their usual therapy or secondary to the beta-blockers. Potential confounders, such as allergen exposure, upper respiratory illness, adjunctive medications, and the severity of the obstructive lung disease were largely ignored. Patients were separated according to asthma and chronic obstructive pulmonary disease (COPD), and according to no, reversible, and irreversible airway obstruction, but the definitions for asthma and COPD were not clearly defined. Patients with COPD and a reversible component greater than 15% were not clearly different than asthmatic patients with a history of smoking. Additionally, the most relevant clinical outcomes, such as peak expiratory flow rates, the number or frequency of asthma attacks, and the subjective sense of wheezing or shortness of breath, were not explored.

Asthma

We found nine placebo-controlled, crossover trials that examined beta-blocker use in asthmatics. Of these, eight were randomized, four had double-blind designs, and three had single-blind designs. Trials examined various beta-blockers, including metoprolol, atenolol, propranolol, labetalol, a nonselective beta-antagonist, and pindolol, an agent with intrinsic sympathomimetic activity.

We found the most consistent results were for propranolol, a nonselective beta-adrenergic antagonist. All four relevant trials showed statistically significant reductions in FEV1 with propranolol compared to placebo.(Tx:L2b) The magnitude of the reductions was 20% in the unblinded[32] and 10% to 25% in the two single-blinded studies,[33, 34] but only 5% or less in the double-blinded study.[35] Because unblinded studies reported greater effects than blinded studies, we suspect measurement bias. We found two randomized, double-blind, placebo controlled trials involving COPD patients that showed significant reductions in FEV1 of 20% to 35% and subjective breathlessness (one study) with propranolol.[36, 37] The latter findings add support for a true adverse effect of propranolol on lung function and symptoms in patients with asthma.

We found two of three relevant placebo controlled trials reported a 5% to 10% decrease in FEV1 and significant decreases in peak expiratory flow rates with metoprolol compared to placebo.[38–40](Tx:L2b) The decrease in FEV1 was statistically significant in only one of the trials.[40] This trial also reported a trend ($p=0.1$) toward significant decreases in the number of asthma-free days in patients assigned to metoprolol compared to those assigned to placebo. Reports of decreased asthma symptoms were largely accounted for by three of 14 study participants. In one of the other small trials, two of 14 patients reported worsening of the frequency and intensity of asthma with metoprolol.[38]

We found one unblinded,[32] two single-blinded,[34, 40] and one double-blinded study,[41] that reported 5% to 10% decreases in FEV1 that were statistically significant in three instances with atenolol compared to placebo or other agents.(Tx:L2b) Two of the trials reported no significant decreases in peak expiratory flow rate.[40, 41] One trial reported no significant increase in the degree of wheeziness, the number of asthma attacks, or the use of inhalant among patients assigned to atenolol.[40] One trial reported significantly less wheeziness and less frequent attacks with atenolol compared to metoprolol.[40]

We found one trial that reported a statistically significant less than 5% decrease in FEV1 with pindolol compared to placebo[35](Tx:L2b) and one that reported a nonsignificant less than 5% decrease in FEV1 with pindolol.[34] (Tx:L2b)We found one trial that reported short-term intravenous, but not long-term oral, labetalol decreased FEV1 by 17% compared to placebo.[33](Tx:L2b)

COPD

We found three randomized double-blind, placebo controlled trials,[36, 37, 42] one randomized single-blind nonplacebo controlled trial,[43] and one randomized, multiple agent trial[6] that examined the use of beta-blockers in COPD. The nonplacebo-controlled trial did not report summary data or statistical analysis, and one of the placebo controlled trials[42] did not quantify exact effects on FEV1.

We found two studies that examined propranolol[37] included patients with only a minimal reversible component of their COPD.[36] The trials reported a statistically significant 19% and 36% ±14% decrease in FEV1, respectively.(Tx:L2b) In one of the trials, participants reported significantly more subjective breathlessness with propranolol compared to metoprolol.[36](Tx:L2b)

We found trials that evaluated metoprolol had mixed results.(Tx:L2b) One[37] reported no statistically significant difference in FEV1 with metoprolol, while the other[36] reported a significant 14 ±20% decrease in FEV1.(Tx:L2b) We doubt the significant decrease in the latter study because the reported standard deviation was larger than the actual point estimate of the effect.

We found trials that evaluated atenolol reported mixed results.(Tx:L2b) Atenolol decreased FEV1 by 14% in one trial, while a second trial reported no significant decreases in FEV1 and no subjective increases in wheeziness or breathlessness with atenolol.[42](Tx:L2b) In one large trial, withdrawal due to bronchospasm was higher for atenolol than captopril (6% versus 0%; $p < 0.0001$).[6](H:L1b)

We found a single study that showed small nonsignificant decreases in FEV1 in patients given intravenous esmolol that was accounted for largely by three patients who were predisposed to bronchospasm by their underlying congestive heart failure.[44](Tx:L2b)

Our practiced judgments

Before using beta-blockers in patients with obstructive lung disease, we consider the reversibility of their respiratory disease and the level of expected additional benefit from beta-blocker treatment compared to other available treatments for hypertension. In patients with hypertension and asthma but no other significant comorbid conditions, we prefer to use proven effective antihypertensive agents other than beta-blockers. In patients with hypertension, asthma, and other conditions where beta-blockers clearly improve survival, such as in postmyocardial infarction patients, we carefully try beta-blockers. We avoid nonselective beta-blockers, such as propranolol, in our asthmatic patients. We prefer beta-1-selective agents and conclude current available best evidence suggests atenolol may be safer than metoprolol.

We routinely use beta-1-selective agents in patients who have COPD and minimally reversible airway disease. We avoid nonselective agents such as propranolol in all of our patients with obstructive lung disease, regardless of the reversibility of their airway disease.

Gout

We identified little high-quality evidence examining the question of whether patients with hypertension who are at risk for gout experience higher rates of clinically apparent gout with diuretics compared to other agents. We found one large trial that reported small excess absolute risks of gout with hydrochlorothiazide compared to placebo (1.7% versus 0.2%, $p<0.05$).[45](H:L1b) We found one large database study from a state within the United States that reported new prescriptions for gout medications, not including NSAIDs, were more common in patients who had also filled prescriptions for diuretics.[46](H:L2c) Specifically, the relative risk for receiving an antigout medication was twice as common in patients taking thiazide diuretics than in those taking nonthiazide antihypertensive agents (relative risk 1.99; 95% CI 1.21 to 3.26).

Our practiced judgments

We avoid thiazide diuretics in patients with frequent or uncontrolled gout.

Incontinence

We found the effect of thiazide diuretics on incontinence has not been well studied. We identified one observational study that examined whether diuretics increased the risk for incontinence among adults over age 60.[47](Tx:L4) There were no differences in continence status between people using and not using diuretics. Among a subset of men who had detrusor instability, however, diuretic use was strongly associated with incontinence (85% versus 25%, $p=0.009$).

Our practiced judgments

In the presence of known incontinence, particularly urge incontinence, we choose an alternative agent to diuretics for initial blood pressure control. We are unclear whether diuretics are good first-line agents in patients at risk for incontinence due to other conditions, such as restricted mobility and moderate to severe dementia. We often prescribe alternative agents for such people.

Left ventricular systolic dysfunction

Alpha-blockers and heart failure

We found one large trial involving hypertensive patients that showed a short acting formulation of an alpha-blocker, doxazosin, increased the incidence of congestive heart failure and did not reduce ischemic events compared to chlorthalidone, a diuretic.[30](Tx:IIb)

Calcium channel blockers and heart failure

Please see earlier section on left ventricular dysfunction for a description of both the potential benefits and harms of various calcium channel blockers for people with known left ventricular systolic dysfunction.

Our practiced judgments

We advise all patients with heart failure due to left ventricular systolic dysfunction to take ACE inhibitors unless they are contraindicated. We also advise patients with stable heart failure symptoms and left ventricular systolic dysfunction to take beta-blockers. We avoid calcium channel blockers other than amlodipine and alpha-blockers in patients with left ventricular systolic dysfunction.

Myocardial infarction

We found two systematic reviews that summarized Level 1 and Level 2 evidence regarding harms of calcium channel blockers in patients with recent myocardial infarction.[48, 49] Both reported suggestive, but inconclusive, findings of increased death and/or reinfarction when various calcium channel blockers, other than amlodipine, were given to patients with recent myocardial infarction and left ventricular dysfunction.

Our practiced judgments

We generally avoid calcium channel blockers, other than amlodipine, in people who have histories of myocardial infarction and left ventricular dysfunction.

 # Which comorbid conditions do not have good indications to avoid specific antihypertensive therapies?

Peripheral vascular disease

Intermittent claudication affects 2% of men and 1% of women over the age of 45.[50] Its prevalence is higher in hypertensive individuals; hypertension has been reported to increase the risk of claudication by 2.4 to 3.9 times.[51]

Although beta-blockers were commonly cited as harmful for patients with claudication, we found a meta-analysis of several randomized controlled trials that showed little or no adverse effects of beta-blockade in peripheral vascular disease patients.[52](Tx:LIa) Pooled analyses of 11 studies involving a total of 127 patients showed no significant reduction in pain-free or maximum walking distances in patients on beta-blocker therapy. Most of the trials compared the effects of up to eight weeks of one or more beta-blockers, including propranolol, metoprolol, acebutolol, atenolol, labetalol, and pindolol with placebo. One small subsequent trial found no difference in walking distance in 49 people with peripheral vascular disease who were treated with atenolol compared with control.[53]

In a large trial involving diabetic people, patients assigned to atenolol were more likely to withdraw due to cold feet or intermittent claudication than those assigned to captopril (4% versus 0%).[6](Tx:LIb) However, the incidence of peripheral vascular disease was higher for patients assigned to captopril (1.6 cases per 1000 patient years) compared to those assigned to atenolol (1.1 cases per 1000 patient years).

Our practiced judgments

We do not avoid beta-blockers in patients with peripheral vascular disease. Because patients with claudication also have high rates of angina and myocardial infarction, we often prefer beta-blockers to diuretics in such patients.

Depression

We found numerous case reports of depression resulting from beta-blocker therapy and several cross-sectional, case-control, cohort, and randomized controlled trials that have reported mixed results with regard to this association. Synthesizing this literature is difficult due to varying definitions of depression, different methods of depression identification, variable comparison groups, and multiple potential confounders such concurrent use of drugs or alcohol.

We found a systematic review that summarized 26 studies published between 1966 and 1996 that addressed associations between beta-blockers and depression.[54] Of these, ten were randomized crossover, cohort, or controlled trials; five compared the effects of beta-blockers to those of placebo. Only two focused primarily on the relationship between beta-blockers and depression.[55, 56] Both used well-validated depression scales to assess the depression diagnosis; both examined the same beta-blockers (atenolol and propranolol); and both found no significant association between beta-blockers and depression.

We found two randomized, double-blind trials that secondarily assessed depression in patients treated with beta-blocker treatment versus nonbeta-blocker treatment.(H:L2b) Results were mixed. One found no relationship between beta-blockers and depression.[57] The other found a significant association between beta-blockers and depression as determined by self or physician report.[58] The positive finding may have occurred by chance alone as multiple statistical tests were performed.

We found a meta-analysis that summarized the prevalence of reported depression in nine of the early hypertension trials that compared beta-blockers and other antihypertensive treatments.[59](H:L2b) No consistent significant associations between beta-blockers and depression were found. The most scientifically rigorous cohort study also concluded that there was no association between beta-blockers and depression.[60](H:L2b)

Our practiced judgments

We conclude current best evidence suggests no causal association between beta-blockers and depression. We do not advise avoidance of beta-blockers in people with depression or history of depression.

Which comorbid conditions have significant clinical trade-offs in prescribing or avoiding specific antihypertensive therapies?

Impotence or sexual dysfunction

We found the effect of diuretics on the incidence of sexual dysfunction was examined in a double-blind trial that randomized 902 men to placebo or one of five antihypertensive drugs. The incidence of erectile dysfunction over two years was higher (16%) among men taking chlorthalidone, a diuretic, than among those taking other agents (3% to 8% for doxazosin, enalapril, amlodipine, and acebutolol) or placebo (5%).[61](H:L1b) About half of the men who reported erectile dysfunction remained on therapy. In women, sexual dysfunction was less common and was not increased for users of diuretics or other agents compared with placebo.

We found a review that summarized three other large randomized, placebo controlled trials that examined the effect of antihypertensive drugs on sexual function.[62](H:L1a) These trials showed approximately two- to threefold higher rates of sexual dysfunction with diuretics compared to placebo. Two of the trials found slightly higher but not statistically significant different rates of sexual dysfunction between people taking a beta-blocker (propranolol or atenolol) and patients taking placebo.

Our practiced judgments

We routinely advise male patients that as many as 15% to 20% of men taking diuretics have sexual dysfunction. We advise them that there are many potential causes of sexual dysfunction and that sexual dysfunction occurring in patients who are taking diuretics can be attributed to the diuretics approximately 50% of the time. We advise patients who have bothersome sexual dysfunction while taking diuretics to try several short periods of discontinuing the diuretic. We prescribe other agents if improvements in sexual function are noted during the short trials of discontinuation. We continue diuretics if no improvements in sexual function are noted during the trials of discontinuation.

Benign prostatic hyperplasia

It is estimated that 12% to 25% of men older than 60 years have benign prostatic hyperplasia (BPH) and concomitant hypertension.[63] We found few studies that specifically investigated the treatment of BPH in patients with hypertension. We found one randomized, double-blind, controlled trial that involved 248 hypertensive men with BPH.[64](Tx:IIb) An alpha-blocker with peripheral effects, doxazosin 4 to 12 mg daily, significantly increased maximum urinary flow rates (2.3 to 3.6 mL/sec) compared with placebo (0.1 mL/sec). Obstructive and irritative symptoms, assessed by a questionnaire, and blood pressure were also significantly reduced with doxazosin compared to placebo. We found another randomized controlled trial that assessed the effects of doxazosin on blood pressure and urinary flow in 232 normotensive and hypertensive men with BPH.[65](Tx:IIb) Compared with placebo, doxazosin, 4 mg daily, significantly reduced blood pressure levels and increased urinary flow rates by about 1 to 2 mL/s.

As previously noted, we found one large trial involving hypertensive patients that showed a short-acting formulation of doxazosin increased the incidence of congestive heart failure and did not reduce ischemic events compared with chlorthalidone, a diuretic.[30](Tx:IIb)

Our practiced judgments

We advise patients with hypertension and BPH that alpha-blockers such as doxazosin will likely improve their BPH symptoms and decrease their blood pressure levels, but that they may also increase the risk of heart disease compared to other agents that treat hypertension. We are uncertain whether such harms represent a class effect of alpha-blockers with peripheral actions. However, because of the possibility of increased rather than decreased cardiovascular harm from alpha-blockers with peripheral effects, we do not routinely choose these agents as drugs of choice for patients with hypertension and BPH. Rather we use antihypertensive agents with proven clinical benefits and seek alternative agents for treating BPH, such as alpha-blockers without peripheral effects (e.g., tamsulosin).

 # Which comorbid conditions have insufficient evidence to either prescribe or avoid specific antihypertensive therapies?

High risk for osteoporotic fractures

We found a meta-analysis of 13 observational studies that examined the relationship between diuretic usage (greater than six months) and the risk of osteoporotic fractures.[66](Tx:L2a) The current use of diuretics was associated with a decrease in the risk of hip fracture (summary odds ratio 0.82; 95% CI 0.73 to 0.91). Short-term use apparently increased fracture risk, while long-term use appeared protective.

Our practiced judgments

We consider data regarding effects of diuretics on osteoporotic fractures insufficient to affect our prescription practices.

Patient Notes

Mr William Lee

- Frequent gouty attacks
- BP 142/86 mm Hg

Recommendations

- Stop HCTZ
- Begin beta-blocker

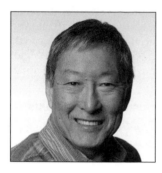

Mrs Marjorie Poindexter

- Frequent migraine headaches
- BP 165/90 mm Hg

Recommendations

- Continue HCTZ
- Add beta-blocker

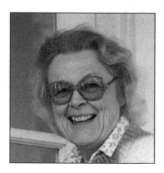

Summary bottom lines

Comorbid conditions with good indications to prescribe specific antihypertensive therapies

- **Angina.** Advise beta-blockers for patients with hypertension and angina. Use long-acting calcium channel blockers if beta-blockers cannot be used or if angina symptoms are uncontrolled despite beta-blocker therapy. Consider concomitant use of ACE inhibitors in high-risk patients with angina and hypertension because they may decrease risk of myocardial infarction and death even though their effects on angina are unclear. (Level 1 evidence)

- **Diabetes.** Advise patients with Type 2 diabetes to take an ACE inhibitor or, alternatively, a beta-blocker or thiazide diuretic. (Level 1 evidence)

- **Diabetes and myocardial infarction.** Advise hypertensive diabetic patients with previous myocardial infarction to take both an ACE inhibitor and a beta-blocker. (Level 1 evidence)

- **Impaired renal function.** Advise ACE inhibitors for patients with mild to moderate impaired renal function and hypertension. (Level 1 evidence)

- **Left ventricular systolic dysfunction.** Advise hypertensive patients with heart failure from systolic dysfunction to take diuretics and ACE inhibitors unless they are contraindicated. Advise patients with stable heart failure from left ventricular systolic dysfunction to take beta-blockers. (Level 1 evidence)

- **Migraines.** Advise hypertensive patients who have frequent migraine headaches that beta-blockers, particularly propranolol and metoprolol, reduce migraine frequency and reduce cardiovascular morbid and mortal events. (Level 1 evidence) Do not preferentially advise clonidine for such patients because its effects on reducing cardiovascular outcomes are not known. (Lacking Level 1 evidence)

- **Myocardial infarction.** Advise beta-blockers without intrinsic sympathomimetic activity for patients with hypertension and myocardial infarction. (Level 1 evidence)

- **Myocardial infarction and asthma.** Carefully try beta-1-selective agents in patients with hypertension and asthma and other conditions where beta-blockers clearly improve survival, such as in postmyocardial infarction patients. (Lack of Level 1 or 2 evidence for significant asthma harm and Level 1 evidence for significant cardiovascular benefits)

- **Myocardial infarction and systolic dysfunction.** Advise concomitant diuretics, beta-blockers, and ACE inhibitors for patients with hypertension and myocardial infarction complicated by left ventricular systolic dysfunction. Titrate beta-blocker doses very slowly and avoid them if patients have acute exacerbations of heart failure symptoms. (Level 1 evidence)

- **Myocardial infarction, systolic dysfunction, and angina.** In patients with hypertension, myocardial infarction, left ventricular systolic dysfunction and symptomatic angina despite ACE inhibitors, beta-blockers, and nitrates, consider adding amlodipine. (Level 2 evidence suggesting no major cardiovascular harms)

- **Perioperative situations.** Consider perioperative beta-blockers for patients with poorly controlled or previously untreated hypertension who are undergoing surgery and have no major contraindications. Consider adding beta-blockers to current medications for patients with well-controlled hypertension and moderate to high cardiac risk who are undergoing surgery and have no contraindications. (Level 1 evidence)

Comorbid conditions without good indications to prescribe specific antihypertensive therapies

- **Lipid abnormalities.** Do not choose specific antihypertensive agents because of potential, yet unproven, adverse clinical effects mediated through lipid levels. Absolute clinical benefits of treating people with moderate to severe hypertension with agents, such as low-dose diuretics and beta-blockers, are likely much larger than any harmful effects mediated through any adverse effects on lipid levels. In patients with mild hypertension, harmful effects of specific antihypertensive agents on lipids could mitigate much of the direct beneficial effects on clinical outcomes, but this latter hypothesis is largely untested. (Lack of Level 1 evidence for clinical cardiovascular benefits)

- **Smokers trying to quit.** Do not advise clonidine as the agent of choice for hypertensive patients who also want to stop smoking. (Lack of Level 1 evidence for clinical cardiovascular benefits)

Comorbid conditions with good indications to avoid specific antihypertensive therapies

- **Asthma.** Avoid nonselective beta-blockers, such as propranolol, in asthmatic patients; when indicated, use beta-1-selective agents, such as atenolol, instead. (Level 2 evidence)

- **COPD.** Avoid nonselective beta-blockers such as propranolol in patients with COPD, regardless of the reversibility of their airway disease. Use beta-1-selective agents in patients who have COPD and minimally reversible airway disease. (Level 2 evidence)

- **Gout.** Avoid thiazide diuretics in patients with frequent or uncontrolled gout. (Level 1 and 2 evidence)
- **Incontinence.** Consider alternative drugs to diuretics in patients with known incontinence, particularly in patients with urge incontinence. (Scant Level 2 evidence)
- **Left ventricular systolic dysfunction.** Avoid calcium channel blockers, other than amlodipine, in patients with left ventricular systolic dysfunction. (Level 2 evidence)
- **Myocardial infarction and systolic dysfunction.** Avoid calcium channel blockers, such as diltiazem, in patients with hypertension, recent myocardial infarction, and left ventricular systolic dysfunction. (Level 2 evidence)

Comorbid conditions without good indications to avoid specific antihypertensive therapies

- **Peripheral vascular disease.** Do not avoid beta-blockers in patients with peripheral vascular disease. (Level 1 evidence)
- **Depression.** Do not avoid beta-blocker therapy in hypertensive patients with depression or history of depression. (Level 1 and 2 evidence)

Comorbid conditions with significant clinical trade-offs in prescribing or avoiding specific antihypertensive therapies

- **Sexual dysfunction.** Advise male patients that as many as 15% to 20% of men taking diuretics have sexual dysfunction. Advise them that there are many potential causes of sexual dysfunction and that sexual dysfunction occurring in patients who are taking diuretics can be attributed to the diuretics approximately 50% of the time. Advise short trials of discontinuation to help sort through whether diuretics are the cause of bothersome sexual dysfunction in particular patients. (Level 1 evidence)
- **Benign prostatic hyperplasia.** Advise patients with hypertension and BPH that alpha-blockers with peripheral actions will likely improve their BPH symptoms and decrease their blood pressure levels but that they may also increase the risk of heart disease compared to other agents that treat hypertension. Because of the possibility of increased rather than decreased cardiovascular harm from alpha-blockers with peripheral effects, choose other antihypertensive agents with proven clinical benefits, and seek alternative agents for treating BPH, such as alpha-blockers, without peripheral effects (e.g., tamsulosin). (Level 1 evidence, albeit lacking class effect evidence)

Comorbid conditions with insufficient evidence to either prescribe or avoid specific antihypertensive therapies

- **Osteoporotic fractures.** Regard data relevant to effects of diuretics on osteoporotic fractures as insufficient to affect prescription practices. (Mixed Level 2 evidence)

> We identified information for this chapter by searching MEDLINE, the Cochrane Controlled Trial Registry and PsycINFO from 1966 to 2000. We searched for English language, human-related literature relevant to multiple specific antihypertensive agents and multiple specific comorbid conditions such as benign prostatic hyperplasia, gout, migraine headaches and myocardial infarction. We screened approximately 800 titles and/or abstracts to help identify the highest quality relevant information to include in this chapter.

References

1. Heidenreich PA, Lee TT, Massie BM. Effect of beta-blockade on mortality in patients with heart failure: a meta-analysis of randomized clinical trials. *J Am Coll Cardiol* 1997; **30**:27-34.

2. Freemantle N, Cleland J, Young P, Mason J, Harrison J. Beta blockade after myocardial infarction: systematic review and meta regression analysis. *BMJ* 1999; **318**:1730-7.

3. Yusuf S, Sleight P, Pogue J, Bosch J, Davies R, Dagenais G. Effects of an angiotensin-converting-enzyme inhibitor, ramipril, on cardiovascular events in high-risk patients. The Heart Outcomes Prevention Evaluation Study Investigators [published erratum appears in *N Engl J Med* 2000; **342**:748]. *N Engl J Med* 2000; **342**:145-53.

4. Garg R, Yusuf S. Overview of randomized trials of angiotensin-converting enzyme inhibitors on mortality and morbidity in patients with heart failure. Collaborative Group on ACE Inhibitor Trials [published erratum appears in *JAMA* 1995; **274**:462]. *JAMA* 1995; **273**:1450-6.

5. Fuller J, Stevens LK, Chaturvedi N, Holloway JF. Antihypertensive therapy for preventing cardiovascular complications in people with diabetes mellitus. (Cochrane Review) In: *The Cochrane Library*, Issue 4, 1997. Oxford: Update Software.

6. UK Prospective Diabetes Study Group. Efficacy of atenolol and captopril in reducing risk of macrovascular and microvascular complications in type 2 diabetes: UKPDS 39. *BMJ* 1998; **317**:713-20.

7. Tatti P, Pahor M, Byington RP, *et al.* Outcome results of the Fosinopril Versus Amlodipine Cardiovascular Events Randomized Trial (FACET) in patients with hypertension and NIDDM. *Diabetes Care* 1998; **21**:597-603.

8. Estacio RO, Jeffers BW, Hiatt WR, Biggerstaff SL, Gifford N, Schrier RW. The effect of nisoldipine as compared with enalapril on cardiovascular outcomes in patients with non-insulin-dependent diabetes and hypertension. *N Engl J Med* 1998; **338**:645-52.

9. Gress TW, Nieto FJ, Shahar E, Wofford MR, Brancati FL. Hypertension and antihypertensive therapy as risk factors for type 2 diabetes mellitus. Atherosclerosis Risk in Communities Study. *N Engl J Med* 2000; **342**:905-12.

10. UK Prospective Diabetes Study Group. Tight blood pressure control and risk of macrovascular and microvascular complications in type 2 diabetes: UKPDS 38 [published erratum appears in *BMJ* 1999; **318**:29]. *BMJ* 1998; **317**:703-13.

11. Lechat P, Packer M, Chalon S, Cucherat M, Arab T, Boissel JP. Clinical effects of beta-adrenergic blockade in chronic heart failure: a meta-analysis of double-blind, placebo-controlled, randomized trials. *Circulation* 1998; **98**:1184-91.

12. Avezum A, Tsuyuki RT, Pogue J, Yusuf S. Beta-blocker therapy for congestive heart failure: a systemic overview and critical appraisal of the published trials. *Can J Cardiol* 1998; **14**:1045-53.

13. Doughty RN, Rodgers A, Sharpe N, MacMahon S. Effects of beta-blocker therapy on mortality in patients with heart failure. A systematic overview of randomized controlled trials. *Eur Heart J* 1997; **18**:560-5.

14. Gheorghiade M, Benatar D, Konstam MA, Stoukides CA, Bonow RO. Pharmacotherapy for systolic dysfunction: a review of randomized clinical trials [published erratum appears in *Am J Cardiol* 1998; **81**:1521]. *Am J Cardiol* 1997; **80**:14H-27H.

15. Packer M, O'Connor CM, Ghali JK, *et al*. Effect of amlodipine on morbidity and mortality in severe chronic heart failure. Prospective Randomized Amlodipine Survival Evaluation Study Group. *N Engl J Med* 1996; **335**:1107-14.

16. Lipton RB, Stewart WF. Prevalence and impact of migraine. *Neurol Clin* 1997; **15**:1-13.

17. Ramadan NM, Schultz LL, Gilkey SJ. Migraine prophylactic drugs: proof of efficacy, utilization and cost. *Cephalalgia* 1997; **17**:73-80.

18. Holroyd KA, Penzien DB, Cordingley GE. Propranolol in the management of recurrent migraine: a meta-analytic review. *Headache* 1991; **31**:333-40.

19. Van De Ven LLM. Age-dependent differences in the efficacy and tolerability of different classes of antihypertensive drugs. *Clin Drug Invest* 1997; **14**:16-22.

20. Solomon GD, Diamond S, Freitag FG. Verapamil in migraine prophylaxis comparison of dosages [abstract]. *Clin Pharmacol Ther* 1987; **41**:202.

21. Solomon GD, Steel JG, Spaccavento LJ. Verapamil prophylaxis of migraine. A double-blind, placebo-controlled study. *JAMA* 1983; **250**:2500-2.

22. Markley HG, Cheronis JC, Piepho RW. Verapamil in prophylactic therapy of migraine. *Neurology* 1984; **34**:973-6.

23. Solomon GD. Verapamil and propranolol in migraine prophylaxis: a double-blind, crossover study [abstract]. *Headache* 1986; **26**:325.

24. Giatras I, Lau J, Levey AS. Effect of angiotensin-converting enzyme inhibitors on the progression of nondiabetic renal disease: a meta-analysis of randomized trials. Angiotensin-Converting-Enzyme Inhibition and Progressive Renal Disease Study Group. *Ann Intern Med* 1997; **127**:337-45.

25. Bakris GL, Weir MR. Angiotensin-converting enzyme inhibitor-associated elevations in serum creatinine: is this a cause for concern? *Arch Intern Med* 2000; **160**:685-93.

26. Mangano DT, Layug EL, Wallace A, Tateo I. Effect of atenolol on mortality and cardiovascular morbidity after noncardiac surgery. Multicenter Study of Perioperative Ischemia Research Group [published erratum appears in *N Engl J Med* 1997; **336**:1039]. *N Engl J Med* 1996; **335**:1713-20.

27. Poldermans D, Boersma E, Bax JJ, *et al*. The effect of bisoprolol on perioperative mortality and myocardial infarction in high-risk patients undergoing vascular surgery. Dutch Echocardiographic Cardiac Risk Evaluation Applying Stress Echocardiography Study Group. *N Engl J Med* 1999; **341**:1789-94.

28. Kasiske BL, Ma JZ, Kalil RS, Louis TA. Effects of antihypertensive therapy on serum lipids. *Ann Intern Med* 1995; **122**:133-41.

29. Grimm RH Jr, Flack JM, Grandits GA, *et al.* Long-term effects on plasma lipids of diet and drugs to treat hypertension. Treatment of Mild Hypertension Study (TOMHS) Research Group. *JAMA* 1996; **275**:1549-56.

30. ALLHAT Collaborative Research Group. Major cardiovascular events in hypertensive patients randomized to doxazosin vs chlorthalidone: the antihypertensive and lipid-lowering treatment to prevent heart attack trial (ALLHAT). *JAMA* 2000; **283**:1967-75.

31. Gourlay SG, Stead LF, Benowitz NL. Clonidine for smoking cessation. (Cochrane Review) In: *The Cochrane Library*, Issue 2, 2000. Oxford: Update Software.

32. Doshan HD, Rosenthal RR, Brown R, Slutsky A, Applin WJ, Caruso FS. Celiprolol, atenolol and propranolol: a comparison of pulmonary effects in asthmatic patients. *J Cardiovasc Pharmacol* 1986; **8**:S105-8.

33. Larsson K. Influence of labetalol, propranolol and practolol in patients with asthma. *Eur J Respir Dis* 1982; **63**:221-30.

34. Benson MK, Berrill WT, Cruickshank JM, Sterling GS. A comparison of four beta-adrenoceptor antagonists in patients with asthma. *Br J Clin Pharmacol* 1978; **5**:415-19.

35. Beumer HM, Teirlinck C, Wiseman RA. Comparative investigation of the respiratory and cardiovascular effect of mepindolol, propranolol and pindolol in asthmatic patients. *Int J Clin Pharmacol Biopharm* 1978; **16**:249-53.

36. Wunderlich J, Macha HN, Wudicke H, Huckauf H. Beta-adrenoceptor blockers and terbutaline in patients with chronic obstructive lung disease. Effects and interaction after oral administration. *Chest* 1980; **78**:714-20.

37. Adam WR, Meagher EJ, Barter CE. Labetalol, beta blockers, and acute deterioration of chronic airway obstruction. *Clin Exp Hypertens* [A] 1982; **4**:1419-28.

38. Hua AS, Assaykeen TA, Nyberg G, Kincaid-Smith PS. Results from a multicentre trial of metoprolol and a study of hypertensive patients with chronic obstructive lung disease. *Med J Aust* 1978; **1**:281-6.

39. Lammers JW, Folgering HT, Van Herwaarden CL. Ventilatory effects of beta 1-receptor-selective blockade with bisoprolol and metoprolol in asthmatic patients. *Eur J Clin Pharmacol* 1984; **27**:141-5.

40. Lawrence DS, Sahay JN, Chatterjee SS, Cruickshank JM. Asthma and beta-blockers. *Eur J Clin Pharmacol* 1982; **22**:501-9.

41. Philip-Joet F, Saadjian A, Bruguerolle B, Arnaud A. Comparative study of the respiratory effects of two beta 1-selective blocking agents atenolol and bevantolol in asthmatic patients. *Eur J Clin Pharmacol* 1986; **30**:13-16.

42. Dorow P, Bethge H, Tonnesmann U. Effects of single oral doses of bisoprolol and atenolol on airway function in nonasthmatic chronic obstructive lung disease and angina pectoris. *Eur J Clin Pharmacol* 1986; **31**:143-7.

43. Clague HW, Ahmad D, Carruthers SG. Influence of cardioselectivity and respiratory disease on pulmonary responsiveness to beta-blockade. *Eur J Clin Pharmacol* 1984; **27**:517-23.

44. Gold MR, Dec GW, Cocca-Spofford D, Thompson BT. Esmolol and ventilatory function in cardiac patients with COPD. *Chest* 1991; **100**:1215-18.

45. Fletcher AE. Adverse treatment effects in the trial of the European Working Party on High Blood Pressure in the Elderly. *Am J Med* 1991; **90**:42S-4S.

46. Gurwitz JH, Kalish SC, Bohn RL, *et al.* Thiazide diuretics and the initiation of anti-gout therapy. *J Clin Epidemiol* 1997; **50**:953-9.

47. Diokno AC, Brown MB, Herzog AR. Relationship between use of diuretics and continence status in the elderly. *Urology* 1991; **38**:39-42.

48. Yusuf S, Furberg CD. Effects of calcium channel blockers on survival after myocardial infarction. *Cardiovasc Drugs Ther* 1987; **1**:343-4.

49. Teo KK, Yusuf S, Furberg CD. Effects of prophylactic antiarrhythmic drug therapy in acute myocardial infarction. An overview of results from randomized controlled trials. *JAMA* 1993; **270**:1589-95.

50. Hughson WG, Mann JI, Garrod A. Intermittent claudication: prevalence and risk factors. *BMJ* 1978; **i**:1379-81.

51. Kannel WB, McGee DL. Update on some epidemiologic features of intermittent claudication: the Framingham Study. *J Am Geriatr Soc* 1985; **33**:13-18.

52. Radack K, Deck C. Beta-adrenergic blocker therapy does not worsen intermittent claudication in subjects with peripheral arterial disease. A meta-analysis of randomized controlled trials. *Arch Intern Med* 1991; **151**:1769-76.

53. Solomon SA, Ramsay LE, Yeo WW, Parnell L, Morris-Jones W. Beta blockade and intermittent claudication: placebo controlled trial of atenolol and nifedipine and their combination. *BMJ* 1991; **303**:1100-4.

54. Ried LD, McFarland BH, Johnson RE, Brody KK. Beta-blockers and depression: the more the murkier? *Ann Pharmacother* 1998; **32**:699-708.

55. Palac DM, Cornish RD, McDonald WJ, Middaugh DA, Howieson D, Bagby SP. Cognitive function in hypertensives treated with atenolol or propranolol. *J Gen Intern Med* 1990; **5**:310-18.

56. Blumenthal JA, Madden DJ, Krantz DS, *et al.* Short-term behavioral effects of beta-adrenergic medications in men with mild hypertension. *Clin Pharmacol Ther* 1988; **43**:429-35.

57. Goldstein G, Materson BJ, Cushman WC, *et al.* Treatment of hypertension in the elderly: II. Cognitive and behavioral function. Results of a Department of Veterans Affairs Cooperative Study. *Hypertension* 1990; **15**:361-9.

58. Veterans Administration Cooperative Study Group on Antihypertensive Agents. Comparison of propranolol and hydrochlorothiazide for the initial treatment of hypertension. II. Results of long-term therapy. *JAMA* 1982; **248**:2004-11.

59. Patten SB. Propranolol and depression: evidence from the antihypertensive trials. *Can J Psychiatry* 1990; **35**:257-9.

60. Gerstman BB, Jolson HM, Bauer M, Cho P, Livingston JM, Platt R. The incidence of depression in new users of beta-blockers and selected antihypertensives. *J Clin Epidemiol* 1996; **49**:809-15.

61. Grimm RH Jr, Grandits GA, Prineas RJ, *et al.* Long-term effects on sexual function of five antihypertensive drugs and nutritional hygienic treatment in hypertensive men and women. Treatment of Mild Hypertension Study (TOMHS). *Hypertension* 1997; **29**:8-14.

62. Prisant LM, Carr AA, Bottini PB, Solursh DS, Solursh LP. Sexual dysfunction with antihypertensive drugs. *Arch Intern Med* 1994; **154**:730-6.

63. Boyle P, Napalkov P. The epidemiology of benign prostatic hyperplasia and observations on concomitant hypertension. *Scand J Urol Nephrol Suppl* 1995; **168**:7-12.

64. Gillenwater JY, Conn RL, Chrysant SG, *et al.* Doxazosin for the treatment of benign prostatic hyperplasia in patients with mild to moderate essential hypertension: a double-blind, placebo-controlled, dose-response multicenter study. *J Urol* 1995; **154**:110-15.

65. Kirby RS. Doxazosin in benign prostatic hyperplasia: effects on blood pressure and urinary flow in normotensive and hypertensive men. *Urology* 1995; **46**:182-6.

66. Jones G, Nguyen T, Sambrook PN, Eisman JA. Thiazide diuretics and fractures: can meta-analysis help? *J Bone Miner Res* 1995; **10**:106-11.

Acknowledgements

We thank Matthew J Bair, MD, for providing the information about alpha-blockers and BPH.

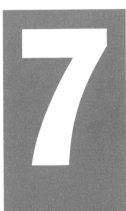

CHAPTER 7

How do we best monitor and facilitate chronic care for patients with hypertension?

Sharon E Straus
David Cherney
Finlay A McAlister
Raj Padwal

What are the best monitoring practices for following patients with hypertension?

How can we predict, assess, and enhance adherence to prescribed therapeutic regimens?

How can we best educate our patients about hypertension and its management?

When is the ideal timing for patient revisits?

Where should we follow-up patients with hypertension?

Who should be involved in follow-up care of patients with hypertension?

How should we manage and monitor patients with hypertensive urgencies and emergencies?

Summary bottom lines

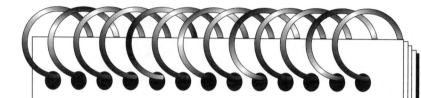

Patient Notes

Mrs Irma Real, age 70, shopkeeper

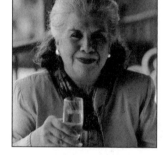

- Smoker: 40 pack years
- Hypertension and angina for 8 years
- Medications: aspirin, metoprolol, and occasional nitroglycerin

Reason for visit

- Recent shortness of breath

Clinical findings

- BP 165/98 mm Hg
- Chest exam: bilateral rales
- Cardiac exam: soft ejection murmur, S3 gallop
- Lower extremity exam 1+edema bilaterally

Clinical question

- What factors should we routinely monitor in follow-up visits for patients with hypertension?

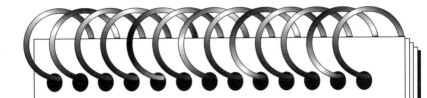

Patient Notes

Mr Dan Taylor, age 51, pharmacist

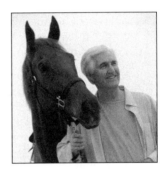

- History of difficult-to-control hypertension that has required three-drug management
- Takes a thiazide, a beta-blocker, and an ACE inhibitor
- Out of medications for a week (forgot to take them on vacation)

Reason for visit

- Afraid his blood pressure is out of control; experiencing headaches

Clinical findings

- BP 200/114 mm Hg
- No symptoms of angina, back pain, heart failure, or stroke
- No papilledema, volume overload, or mental status changes

Clinical question

What is the treatment of choice for an adult patient with a "hypertensive urgency" precipitated by forgetting to take his medicines?

What are the best monitoring practices for following patients with hypertension?

Although multiple guidelines give consensus-based recommendations regarding hypertension management, the actual care that hypertensive patients receive is highly variable and does not always result in controlled blood pressure.[14] Retrospective chart reviews and cross-sectional surveys document that large numbers of hypertensive patients have inadequate blood pressure control.[5-8] Audits suggest that many clinicians do not routinely search for concomitant cardiac risk factors in patients with hypertension and that patients do not always receive information on lifestyle modification.[5,9,10] For example, a cross-sectional survey of 2676 patients with mild to moderate hypertension showed that 98% had at least one additional risk factor for cardiovascular disease.[11] Of these, only 38% recalled receiving information about smoking cessation, and 38% remembered receiving advice about exercise.

This chapter addresses various approaches for monitoring and managing patients with hypertension and the evidence that underpins these approaches. We found no evidence that compared the utility or cost-effectiveness of different comprehensive monitoring strategies for patients with hypertension. Specifically, we were unable to find any studies that determined what elements should comprise the optimal follow-up encounter for a patient with hypertension. Therefore, much of what follows are our practiced approaches that rely only indirectly on research evidence.

Goals of follow-up visits

We use our own expertise, combined with our patients' unique values and circumstances, and the best available evidence to help decide the content of individual patients' follow-up visits. Most often, we monitor the items outlined in Box 7.1.

Box 7.1. Suggested aims for follow-up visits.

- Assess whether blood pressure is at target level
- Screen for complications of hypertension (target organ damage)
- Assess and treat comorbid cardiovascular risk factors
- Assess relevant comorbid illnesses and therapies
- Query about adverse effects of prescribed therapies
- Evaluate adherence to lifestyle and therapeutic recommendations
- Ask about psychosocial circumstances, preferences and values

Target blood pressure levels

As discussed in Chapter 3, multiple prognostic studies establish that there is a continuous, strong graded relationship between blood pressure level and adverse cardiovascular outcomes.(Pr: LI) As discussed in Chapter 4, several large randomized trials prove that antihypertensive drug therapy decreases cardiovascular morbidity and mortality in people with hypertension.(Tx: LI) It is not clear whether the decreases in morbidity and mortality are directly related to the blood pressure lowering effects of the antihypertensive agents or to their other heterogeneous effects. Regardless of this imperfect knowledge, we use blood pressure levels as surrogate measures for monitoring response to therapy.

We found no clear threshold blood pressure level that separates people who will and will not suffer adverse cardiovascular outcomes. Trials described in Chapters 4 and 6 generally have titrated therapeutic regimens to achieve systolic levels of less than 140 to 160 mm Hg and diastolic levels of less than 90 to 95 mm Hg. Trials involving patients with diabetes and/or renal disease have titrated therapeutic regimens to lower diastolic levels of less than 80 to 85 mm Hg.

We found controversy regarding whether lowering blood pressure too much, particularly diastolic levels, increases cardiovascular risk in a so-called J-curve effect. Some observational studies show higher mortality rates in people with diastolic blood pressure levels below 75 to 85 mm Hg.[12,13] This is not surprising because extremes in any continuous variable, such as blood pressure, are likely to be incompatible with good health. The clinical question of interest is not whether individuals with low diastolic blood pressure have higher mortality rates. Rather, we want to know whether aggressive lowering of blood pressure in hypertensive patients results in poorer outcomes compared with less aggressive management.[14]

Table 7.1 shows results of some of the studies that have examined the J-curve effect. It is arranged by the study designs that are most (case series) to least (randomized trials) likely to be susceptible to biases. Studies with weaker designs tend to suggest stronger J-curve relationships, whereas randomized trials suggest no or little J-curve effects. Moreover, none of the trials that specifically compare aggressive lowering of blood pressure with less aggressive lowering report adverse J-curve effects.[15,16,17](Tx: LIb) Aggressive lowering of blood pressure in these trials is variously defined as less than 150 mm Hg systolic and/or less than 80 to 85 mm Hg diastolic.

Table 7.1. The strength of the J-curve association in relation to study design.

Reference	Study design	Strength of association[a] (95% confidence intervals)
Stewart[12]	Case series	Relative risk 5.4 (1.6 to 18.7)
Merlo et al.[18]	Cohort	Relative risk 1.7 (0.8 to 3.6)
Cooper et al.[19]	Subgroup of randomized trial	Relative risk 1.5 (not provided)
Hansson et al.[16]	Randomized controlled trial	Relative risk 1.1 (0.9 to 1.3)

[a]Refers to the comparison of event rates in participants with lowest treated diastolic blood pressure and referent categories.

On the other hand, trials demonstrate fewer adverse cardiovascular outcomes among hypertensive diabetic people randomized to aggressive blood pressure lowering, compared to less aggressive blood pressure lowering, but no differences in outcomes among people who do not have diabetes.[15-17](Tx: LIb)

Our practiced judgments

We conclude that there are likely neither major benefits nor major harms associated with lowering blood pressure below 140/85 mm Hg. If patients have diabetes, we aim for lower target levels of less than 130 to 135 mm Hg systolic and less than 75 to 80 mm Hg diastolic.

Complications of hypertension (target organ damage)

We did not identify any prospective studies that assessed the precision and accuracy of the follow-up clinical examination for detecting target organ damage. Likewise, we did not find any prospective studies that evaluated the clinical impact of routine monitoring for particular target organ damage.

What experts recommend

We summarize consensus recommendations from various expert guidelines regarding routine follow-up examinations in Tables 7.2 and 7.3.[14, 20-23]

Table 7.2. Example consensus recommendations regarding initial physical examination in hypertensive individuals.

Examination maneuver	Our comment
Blood pressure level	Clearly related to cardiovascular risk
Fundoscopic examination	Reliability, accuracy and utility not established
Palpate for sustained cardiac apex beat	Accuracy and utility not established
Jugular venous pressure for volume overload	Fair accuracy when combined with other findings[24, 25]
Chest examination for volume overload (rales)	Fair reliability, fair accuracy when combined with other findings[24]
Cardiac examination for systolic dysfunction (S3)	Fair reliability, fair accuracy when combined with other findings[24]
Cardiac examination for valvular heart disease	Fair accuracy[26]
Peripheral pulses for volume and bruits	Unclear accuracy
Neurologic examination for occult cerebrovascular disease	Reliability and utility not established

Table 7.3. Example consensus recommendations regarding initial laboratory tests in hypertensive individuals.

Tests	Our comment
Urinalysis	Specificity for detecting target organ damage unclear
Serum creatinine	Specificity for detecting target organ damage unclear but thought high
Chest radiograph for determining volume overload and/or enlarged heart	Fair accuracy when combined with other findings[24]
Electrocardiogram	Fair accuracy for ischemia and left ventricular hypertrophy
Serum fasting glucose	Clearly related to cardiovascular risk
Lipid profile including total, LDL, and HDL cholesterol	Clearly related to cardiovascular risk
Serum sodium	Predictive value for secondary causes of hypertension unclear, utility unclear
Serum potassium	Predictive value for secondary causes of hypertension unclear, but thought useful

What we do

We routinely ask our patients about chest pain, shortness of breath, episodic dizziness, weakness, blurred vision, slurred speech, memory loss, cognitive function, and leg pain. If answers to such screening questions suggest cardiac dysfunction or volume overload, we check for elevated jugular venous pressure, pulmonary rales, heart murmurs or gallops, and peripheral edema on physical examination. If answers to our screening questions suggest orthostasis, we assess supine and standing blood pressure. We perform focused neurological examinations, including mental status examinations in people who report symptoms suggesting transient ischemic attack or stroke. We vary in our practices regarding measuring ankle/arm indices for diagnosis of peripheral vascular disease. Some of us reserve this physical examination maneuver for patients with leg pain; others favor more routine testing for peripheral vascular disease because its presence may affect our abilities to prognosticate.

We routinely check urinalyses and serum creatinine levels in our hypertensive patients because results of these tests may affect our ability to prognosticate and also affect our treatment choices (see Chapters 3, 4 and 6). For example, we might test for microalbuminuria in patients whose estimated cardiovascular risk is borderline because the presence of microalbuminuria in such patients helps us determine whether or not to recommend treatment. We also routinely check serum potassium levels to monitor potential adverse effects of diuretics and/or ACE inhibitors. We were unable to identify any evidence that proscribes the appropriate interval for periodic screening of electrolytes and creatinine when diuretics and ACE inhibitors are prescribed.

What we don't do

Although approximately 10% of hypertensive people may have retinopathy,[27](Level 3b) we found traditional fundoscopy examination for retinopathy had questionable reliability. Developed in 1939, the Keith-Wegener-Barker classification for grading hypertensive retinopathy includes assessing arteriolar narrowing, focal arteriolar constriction, arteriovenous crossing, hemorrhage and exudates, and disc edema.[28] Such retinal signs also may be seen in people without hypertension, and we are unsure of their accuracy in clinical practice.[27] Interrater reliability for detecting hypertensive retinopathy appears poor.[29, 30] In one study, a panel of two general physicians and two ophthalmologists, who were unaware of the patients' clinical status, examined 25 consecutive untreated patients from a hospital hypertension clinic.[30](Dx: L2b) Direct ophthalmoscopy and fundal photographs were used to assess retinopathy using the Keith-Wegener-Barker grading system. The coefficient of variation between observers was 38%. Because we do not trust our own abilities to reliably or accurately detect hypertensive retinopathy, and such findings would not affect our treatment choices, most of us do not routinely perform fundoscopy in our hypertensive patients.

We do not routinely obtain laboratory investigations, such as thyroid testing, complete blood counts, and serum calcium in our initial and follow-up assessments of hypertensive individuals because they are not useful for assessing either cardiovascular risk or target organ damage.

What we selectively do

We do not routinely obtain chest radiographs in all of our hypertensive patients. However, we do use this test to help determine cardiomegaly and volume overload in selected patients who have other symptoms or signs suggestive of cardiac target organ damage. Although many national guidelines suggest routine electrocardiograms (ECGs) for detecting cardiac target organ damage in patients with hypertension, we found no evidence that showed performing routine ECGs impacts management or patient outcomes or is cost effective.[1-3](Dx: L5) We use this test selectively in people who have symptoms suggestive of ischemia or symptoms and physical examination findings suggestive of arrhythmia.

We occasionally use echocardiography, a more sensitive but more expensive test than electrocardiography, to help detect either asymptomatic left ventricular systolic dysfunction or left ventricular hypertrophy. We reserve this test for patients who already have evidence of cardiac target organ damage, such as those with a history or electrocardiogram suggestive of past myocardial infarction or for patients who have borderline estimated risks for cardiovascular disease.

Comorbid cardiovascular risk factors

We periodically reassess and treat comorbid cardiovascular risk factors, such as lipid abnormalities, diabetes, tobacco abuse, obesity, and physical inactivity, in all of our hypertensive patients. We did not find high quality evidence regarding the appropriate periodicity of such reassessments.

Comorbid illnesses and therapies

We were unable to find any prospective studies that described which comorbid conditions were worth routinely monitoring. In Chapter 6, we discussed how the presence of particular comorbid conditions could influence our choice of antihypertensive therapy. For example, if a patient who had been maintained on a thiazide diuretic developed frequent migraines or ischemic coronary artery disease, we would consider switching therapy to a beta-blocker. If a hypertensive patient develops severe dementia and becomes incapacitated, we might discuss discontinuing therapy with the patient and family as the goals of therapy might be different now than at the onset of antihypertensive therapy. Box 7.2 lists comorbid conditions that we routinely note because they may affect particular antihypertensive treatment choices.

Box 7.2. Comorbid conditions that could affect treatment choices.

- Angina
- Benign prostatic hypertrophy
- Dementia
- Diabetes
- Gout
- Incontinence
- Left ventricular systolic dysfunction
- Migraine headaches
- Myocardial infarction
- Obstructive airway disease
- Sexual dysfunction

We also routinely review other medications that our patients are taking, including both prescription and over-the-counter medications. For information regarding medications that interfere with blood pressure, see Chapter 8.

Adverse effects

Between 10% and 18% of people receiving antihypertensive therapy experience some type of adverse effect.[31] When surveyed, patients frequently say they want information about adverse effects of therapy, but they do not often receive it.[32,33] In a survey of 623 patients receiving hypertensive medications, 41% reported adverse drug effects, and only 31% were satisfied with the amount of information they received about these effects.[33]

Adverse drug effects can worsen a patient's quality of life and may lead to noncompliance.[34] No good data suggest the best way to identify an adverse drug reaction. One study observed that a symptom questionnaire elicited from patients a higher frequency of adverse effects than did an interview.[31]

Adverse effects vary by classes of agents and by agents within classes. For example, diuretic therapy can cause hypokalemia, hyponatremia, prerenal azotemia, and sexual dysfunction; ACE inhibitors can cause cough; beta-blockers can cause bradycardia and fatigue; calcium channel blockers can cause constipation and peripheral edema; and peripheral alpha-blockers can cause nasal stuffiness and dizziness.

Our practiced judgments

We routinely ask open-ended questions of our patients regarding difficulties with medications. Some of us ask specific questions related to adverse effects that occur frequently, such as sexual dysfunction with diuretics and cough with ACE inhibitors. We routinely use electronic drug formularies to help sort out specific adverse effects.

Reinforcement of healthy lifestyles and self-care techniques

We follow clinical practice guidelines that suggest that clinicians should reinforce nonpharmacological advice during follow-up visits.[1,3] For example, we use follow-up visits to reinforce moderation of alcohol and sodium intake, avoidance of tobacco, active physical lifestyles and healthy diets. We advise patients to monitor their pressure between office visits. Although we realize there is little proof regarding the efficacy of such routine counseling, we believe the absence of evidence is not proof that there is no benefit to doing any of these.

Social circumstances, preferences, and values

We routinely enquire about our patient's social circumstances, including their type of employment, social support, and living circumstances. We encourage patients to be involved in their own health care, and we try to ascertain their preferences about particular types of care and follow-up approaches.

How can we predict, assess, and enhance adherence to prescribed therapeutic regimens?

We use the terms "adherence" or "compliance" to describe the extent to which patients follow instructions that are given for prescribed therapies. We do not intend the terms to be judgmental or paternalistic. Plainly stated, potential benefits of negotiated therapeutic regimens are negated when patients either cannot or do not adhere to them. Patients who are more adherent to their antihypertensive regimen are more likely to achieve blood pressure control than patients who are less adherent.[35] Noncompliance with antihypertensive regimens has been linked to increased hospitalization rates in one case-control study. [36](E: L3b)

Aside from clinical trials, usual compliance with prescribed medications is approximately 50% for both short- and long-term regimens (range of 0 to 100%), and there is considerable variation from week to week.[37-39] Survey data suggest that adherence to medication regimens is better than adherence to nonpharmacological therapy.[40, 41] Thresholds of adherence necessary to achieve clinical therapeutic benefits are not really known, but 80% compliance with prescribed antihypertensive regimens has been reported as necessary to achieve expected reductions in blood pressure.[42](Tx: IIb)

Predicting adherence

We did not find consistent high quality evidence or a systematic review that identified the most important predictors of adherence. Various predictors of poor compliance that have been reported include particular cultural health beliefs, complex medication regimens, experience with adverse effects, recent diagnosis of hypertension, and poor social support. [40, 43–51](Generally Pr: L3 or lower) Magnitudes of reported associations between factors and poor compliance generally were modest, and most associations were not replicated in multiple studies.

Nonattendance at appointments and loss of responsiveness to a previously adequate dose of treatment can be clues that patients are noncompliant.[43](Pr: IIa) Patients' response to therapy is only weakly related to compliance.[42](Pr: IIb) Relationships between compliance and adverse effects have not been studied extensively. Among patients prescribed diuretics for the treatment of hypertension, reductions in serum potassium were sensitive (82%) but not specific (48%) for ruling out noncompliance.[42]

Assessing adherence

Some evidence suggests that clinicians have difficulty evaluating compliance in their patients. In one study, primary care physicians were asked to estimate compliance among patients they knew well. The sensitivity of clinical judgment for detecting noncompliance was only 10%.[52] A survey of physicians and patients confirmed that physicians tended to overestimate compliance.[47]

Physicians can use several methods to measure compliance. When choosing one, consider the perceived threat to the patient's autonomy and his or her preferences. In clinical practice, self-report of medication adherence is the method most readily available, and a meta-analysis of four high-quality studies that compared self-report with other compliance measures suggests that it is fairly reliable.[43](Dx: IIa) A positive response to a single, nonthreatening question, "Have you ever missed any of your pills?" was associated with a likelihood ratio of 4.4 for noncompliance. The likelihood ratio for a negative test result when patients reported they were compliant was 0.5.

Clinicians also can perform direct measurements of either drug or metabolite levels or of tracer compounds. They can count pills, although this practice may overestimate compliance rates.[53] They can check pharmacy records for prescription refills, although we found no evidence that measuring compliance with pharmacy records is accurate. They can also use medication event monitors or electronically tagged pill dispensers.[54-56] Currently, this system is not easily incorporated into the average practice because of its cost and lack of availability. An additional limitation is that opening the bottle does not mean the patient has taken the medicine. Finally, physicians can confirm compliance by directly observing patients taking medications and measuring blood pressure. This method has the potential to cause severe hypotension if the patient has been truly noncompliant.[57]

Enhancing adherence

Compliance with medical recommendations is a complex challenge. The rationale for improving adherence is based on the premise that our patients will have better outcomes if they follow appropriate medical recommendations. Increased adherence is not an appropriate outcome by itself; attempts to increase compliance should be judged by their effects on clinical outcomes.

We identified a review that summarized high quality randomized controlled trials of interventions to change medication adherence in which both compliance and treatment effects were measured.[58](Tx: LIa) These trials had 80% or greater follow-up rates; trials with hypertensive participants were at least six months in duration.

We summarized the seven interventions that have been tested in patients with hypertension in Table 7.4.[59-65] Most of these trials assessed compliance by self-report and pill counts; two trials also performed spot checks of drug levels in the urine.[61, 65] None of the trials measured significant clinical endpoints, such as cardiovascular events. While the results of the trials suggested that complex compliance regimens were more effective than simple ones, data were relatively scant and the cost effectiveness of more versus less intensive adherence strategies was not clearly established.

Table 7.4. Trial evidence about interventions to improve medication adherence.

Participants:	267 patients with hypertension.[59]
Intervention:	Automated telephone patient monitoring and educational and motivational counseling versus usual medical care.
Outcome:	Improved medication adherence (18% intervention versus 12% control; $p=0.03$) and significant decrease in diastolic blood pressure in adjusted analyses.
Participants:	457 patients with newly diagnosed hypertension.[60]
Intervention:	Worksite care managed by trained nurses using standard protocols versus usual care by patients' own physicians.
Outcome:	Both medication adherence and blood pressure control were significantly improved in the intervention group (mean reduction in diastolic blood pressure at one year was 12.1 +/–0.6 mm Hg versus 6.5 +/–0.6 mm Hg; $p <0.001$).
Participants:	389 patients with mild to moderate hypertension.[61]
Intervention:	Once daily versus twice daily metoprolol.
Outcome:	Adherence improved significantly with once-daily use of metoprolol; no effect on blood pressure control.
Participants:	191 patients with poorly controlled hypertension.[62]
Intervention:	Antihypertensive medications given in traditional pill vials versus special blister packaging format.
Outcome:	No difference between two groups in either compliance or control; blister packaging perceived as difficult and inconvenient.
Participants:	136 patients with newly diagnosed hypertension.[63]
Intervention:	Self-recording of blood pressure and monthly home visits versus self-recording of blood pressure versus monthly home visits alone versus neither self-recorded blood pressure nor home visits.
Outcome:	No significant differences between any groups in medication compliance or blood pressure control. In patients who said they had trouble remembering to take their pills, both self-recording and home visits improved blood pressure control.
Participants:	38 noncompliant men who were not at goal blood pressure.[60]
Intervention:	Self-monitoring of blood pressure, charting measurements and pill-taking, bimonthly reinforcement from research assistant, and rewards for improvements versus usual care.
Outcome:	Significant improved compliance and trend toward better blood pressure control in the intervention group compared with the control group.
Participants:	134 untreated hypertensive men.
Intervention:	Care at worksite by occupational health physicians versus detailed education about hypertension and adherence versus both care at worksite and education versus usual care.[65]
Outcome:	No significant differences in medication adherence or blood pressure control.

How can we best educate our patients about hypertension and its management?

Several studies on patient education interventions to improve blood pressure control have produced mixed results, suggesting the need for a rigorous, up-to-date systematic review. Measuring important clinical outcomes, not just patient knowledge, would strengthen future studies. For example, one study of an education intervention increased patient knowledge about hypertension, but there was no associated improvement in blood pressure control.[65](Tx: IIb)

In another study, 287 patients with newly diagnosed hypertension were randomized to receive an educational intervention or usual care.[66] The intervention group received an educational booklet that described hypertension and its management, two group educational talks, and one tutorial meeting, to which their relatives also were invited to attend. During group sessions, participants were told about hypertension, its management, pharmacological treatment and adherence to medications and appointments. Dietitians also talked about salt restriction, weight control, and alcohol moderation. One month later, they received a personal tutorial meeting to discuss individual issues. After six months, both groups reduced their blood pressure significantly, but there were no differences noted between the intervention and control groups. The intervention group was able to complete more correct answers on the hypertension questionnaire than the control group. Only 40% of the intervention group attended one or more educational sessions.

A systematic review of studies investigating the effects of psychoeducational care on blood pressure identified 89 randomized or quasirandomized studies.[67](Tx: IIa) Blood pressure decreased significantly with psychoeducational care. However, the authors provided little detail about what comprised the individual interventions or the validity of the individual studies. Interactive computerized patient education systems were the subject of another systematic review of trials that included one intervention for hypertensive patients.[68, 69] This trial involving hypertensive patients measured patient knowledge about hypertension rather than clinical outcomes.[69]

Our practiced judgments

We conclude that the best psychoeducational care for patients with hypertension is not known. We also conclude that the best methods for maximizing adherence to therapeutic regimens are not known. We think the suggestions outlined in Box 7.3 represent one commonsense approach.

Box 7.3. Suggestions for healthcare professionals to educate patients about hypertension and improve adherence.

- Provide patients with written and verbal instructions regarding the etiology and prognosis of hypertension, as well as the benefits of pharmacological and nonpharmacological therapy. Provide information at their reading level.

- Simplify medication regimens. Attempt to prescribe medications that can be taken once a day, whenever possible. Suggest appropriate behavior strategies, such as tailoring pill-taking to patients' daily habits and rituals. Advocate self-monitoring of medication adherence and blood pressure.

- Try to choose medications that are: realistically priced from the patient's perspective; not likely to produce adverse effects that are particularly bothersome to the individual patient; and tailored to the individual's specific mix of comorbid cardiovascular risk factors, target organ damage, and coincident comorbid conditions (See Chapters 4, 5 and 6).

 # When is the ideal timing for patient revisits?

Revisit intervals

We found little guidance to help clinicians decide on the appropriate timing for follow-up visits. We were not able to find any high quality trials that evaluated what factors are useful in setting visit intervals or most importantly, whether the frequency of visits influenced the control of blood pressure. Factors that clinicians may want to consider in deciding about the revisit interval include the severity and variability of the blood pressure, the complexity of the medication regimen and the patients' adherence to it, and the patients' need for ongoing nonpharmacological advice.

Several studies that surveyed primary care clinicians to determine their revisit intervals for hypothetical patient scenarios identified significant variability, ranging from 1 to 48 weeks.[70-72] Characteristics of the patient, the physician, and the current visit may determine revisit intervals.[73] For example, the interval may be shorter if a patient is thought to be sicker, or if a medication is started or changed, or a test is ordered. One study looked at the revisit interval for 164 patients with an established diagnosis of hypertension, diabetes mellitus, angina, or musculoskeletal pain.[73] Investigators interviewed the 11 primary care physicians who provided ongoing care for these patients and found substantial variation in the revisit intervals. When physicians perceived the patient to be in poor or fair health, the revisit interval was seven weeks, while for patients perceived to be in good or excellent health, the interval was 13 weeks. All physicians lengthened revisit intervals for routine visits and shortened them when changing management.

Optimal timing for medication titration

Randomized trials have used various protocols for titrating antihypertensive medications ranging from every two weeks to several months. We identified one randomized, open-label trial in which the investigators attempted to evaluate the optimal timing for drug titration in hypertensive patients.[74](Tx: L2b) Nearly 3 000 hypertensive patients were randomized to either slow titration or fast titration with quinapril. The slow group received clinic visits at 6, 12, and 18 weeks; the fast group's visits occurred at two, four, and six weeks. Both groups were initially given quinapril 20 mg/day. If blood pressure did not normalize at less than 140/90 mm Hg, the dose was titrated to 40 mg daily and then 80 mg daily. The quinapril dose was immediately doubled if systolic blood pressure was higher than 220 mm Hg and/or diastolic blood pressure was higher than 115 mm Hg at any visit.

Significantly more people in the slow titration group achieved blood pressure control than in the fast group. This was true at one month (NNT 14; 95% CI 9 to 17) and at three months (NNT 17; 95% CI 19 to 62). Although there was no difference between the two groups in the proportion of people who experienced an adverse event, the slow titration group experienced fewer severe adverse events. Limitations to this study included low rates of follow-up. By the third visit, only 65% of the people remained in the slow titration group and 75% in the fast titration group; the high dropout rate was not explained.

Consensus guidelines for revisit intervals

Several national clinical practice guidelines for hypertension management have addressed the issue of revisit frequency. They are summarized in Table 7.5.

Table 7.5. Suggested guidelines for revisit intervals.

Monthly	• For pharmacological therapy until two blood pressure readings are below the target.
	• Newly-diagnosed patient seen one to two months after initiation of therapy. Determine adequacy of blood pressure control, degree of patient adherence and presence of adverse effects.
3 months	• Treatment and blood pressure stable.
	• For patients with symptoms, severe hypertension, intolerance of medications, other cardiovascular risk factors or target organ damage.
3 to 6 months	• Stable blood pressure.
	• For nonpharmacological interventions.
	• For pharmacological therapy, when target blood pressure is reached.
6 months	• Maximum revisit interval.

Our practiced judgments

We have variable opinions but tend to follow patients with severe hypertension or patients in whom we are titrating therapy every few weeks. We follow patients with controlled hypertension at two- to six-month intervals, depending upon their mix and severity of comorbid illness.

 # Where should we follow-up patients with hypertension?

Although traditionally patients with hypertension are monitored through regular doctor visits, alternative methods of managing patients have been evaluated. In this section, we describe the success of the following models of care: patient-directed-home-hypertension management, hypertension specialty care clinics, and telephone monitoring.

Self-directed management

We found one small trial that evaluated patient-directed-home-hypertension management. An unblinded study randomized 31 patients with stable hypertension to a patient-directed management group or usual care.[75](Tx: L2b) The primary outcome measure was whether the daytime mean arterial blood pressure changed over an eight-week period, as shown by ambulatory blood pressure monitoring.

In the patient-directed group, participants learned the technique of home blood pressure monitoring. They were told to increase their medication in a stepwise fashion using an algorithm when their blood pressure remained above 160 mm Hg systolic or 95 mm Hg diastolic for a two-week period.[75] The algorithm also specified decreasing therapy when blood pressure less than 110 mm Hg systolic and less than 70 mm Hg diastolic lasted more than one week. In the usual care group, a physician adjusted antihypertensive therapy according to standardized guidelines that did not specify visit frequency.

In the patient-directed group, daytime mean arterial pressure decreased by 0.1 mm Hg. In the usual care group, it increased by 1.9 mm Hg (p=0.04). The total number of physician visits was significantly greater in the patient-directed management group (1.1 versus 0.2 physician visits per participant per eight weeks; p = 0.05) than in the usual care group. There were no differences in the number of antihypertensive medications used between the two groups.

Hypertension clinics

We found two prospective studies that evaluated whether hypertension clinics are effective. In one, 831 newly diagnosed patients were allocated to their general practitioner or a hypertension clinic.[76](Tx: L2b) No difference was found in survival between the two groups after a median follow-up of 11 years.

A single-blind, randomized study compared three models of care: a specialized blood pressure clinic at a hospital, an independent nurse practitioner clinic, and a shared care clinic in which general practitioners and hospital specialists shared patient management in a formal manner.[77](Tx: L1b) After two years of follow-up, blood pressure control was similar in all three groups. The participant dropout rate was 3% in the shared care group, 14% in the hospital clinic, and 9% in the nurse-practitioner clinic. Almost half of patients and almost 70% of general practitioners preferred shared care of follow-up. While researchers touted shared care as more cost effective than either the clinic care or nurse-practitioner care, there were minor problems with the economic analysis. The model did not include patients with poorly controlled blood pressure, who presumably are more expensive to treat, nor noncompliant patients. Nor did the model include a sensitivity analysis.

Telephone monitoring

We found one trial that evaluated effects of telephone monitoring and counseling. An interactive computer-based telecommunication system that conversed with patients in their homes between office visits was compared to a control intervention in 267 patients. The computer asked questions over the phone and gave feedback to promote medication adherence. Patients communicated using the touch-tone keypad on their telephone. The telecommunication system increased medication adherence and significantly decreased diastolic blood pressure after adjustment for multiple factors.[59](Tx: L1b)

Our practiced judgments

We have varying access to different resources to help monitor patients with hypertension. We routinely see patients in our primary care clinics; some of us work with nurse practitioners and physician assistants to help ensure "adequate" follow-up care.

Who should be involved in follow-up care of patients with hypertension?

We located studies about three different groups of health care professionals to help follow patients with hypertension: nurses, pharmacists, and physician-pharmacist teams.

Nurses

We found one trial that showed patients benefit from nurse counseling to reduce alcohol consumption, dietary fat, salt intake, and weight; to stop smoking; and to increase physical activity.[78](Tx: LIb) At 18 weeks of follow-up, participants who received low-level counseling showed significant decreases in alcohol and salt intake compared to those in a control group. Patients who received high-level counseling showed improved blood pressure control compared to patients in the control group.

Pharmacists

We located one systematic review that evaluated the effects of expanding outpatient pharmacists' roles on health services utilization, costs of health services, and patient outcomes.[79](Tx: LIa) One study in the review assessed the pharmacist's role in the care of hypertensive patients with diabetes mellitus and/or hypertension from a primary care clinic.[80](Tx: LIb) Patients were randomized to usual care or to pharmacist management of their drug therapy. The pharmacist prescribed medications and modified therapy based on the patient response. No change in blood pressure was noted between the two groups.

In the second small study of a community pharmacy intervention, patients were allocated alternately to either usual care or monthly meetings with a pharmacist that offered counseling on diet, exercise, and medication use. [81](Tx: L2b) The experimental group showed an increase in blood pressure control. This small study from a single practice was not randomized, and the counseling was delivered by a single pharmacist who was also one of the investigators.

Physician-pharmacist teams

We identified a small, controlled, single-blind study that assessed whether a physician-pharmacist team achieved blood pressure control in patients with uncontrolled hypertension.[82](Tx: LIb) Ninety-five patients with uncontrolled hypertension were assigned to usual care or to physician-pharmacist care based on whether the last digit of their social security numbers were even or odd. In the intervention group, the pharmacist interacted with patients at each visit and made recommendations to physicians about cost of medications, performing laboratory monitoring, initiating new medications, and increasing drug dosages. The same physicians cared for patients in the intervention group and control group, possibly contaminating the results. At six months, more people in the intervention group achieved blood pressure control than in the control group (NNT 3; 95% CI 1 to 5). The pharmacists made 162 recommendations; physicians declined 7.4% of them.

Our practiced judgments

We have varying access to different resources to help monitor patients with hypertension. We routinely see patients in our primary care clinics and work with both nurses and pharmacists to help ensure "adequate" follow-up care.

How should we manage and monitor patients with hypertensive urgencies and emergencies?

Definitions

In a hypertensive emergency, a patient has evidence of target organ damage, such as encephalopathy, unstable angina, stroke, or a dissecting aortic aneurysm. The absolute level of blood pressure in this situation is not as important as the evidence of end organ damage.[83] In a hypertensive urgency, the blood pressure is elevated, but there is no evidence of end organ damage.

Treatment for hypertensive emergencies

We found guidelines for managing hypertensive emergency that suggested that the mean arterial blood pressure be reduced by less than or equal to 25% within two hours and to 160/100 mm Hg by six hours.[2,3] Avoiding excessive reduction in blood pressure was advised because this can precipitate renal, cerebral, or coronary ischemia. Frequent monitoring of blood pressure responses to treatment, every 15 to 30 minutes, was also recommended.

We were unable to identify any prospective studies that addressed the questions of how quickly blood pressure should be controlled in a hypertensive emergency or when maintenance therapy should begin. We identified three small trials that compared various therapies in patients with hypertensive emergencies (Table 7.6).[84–86](Tx: L2b) The three trials used different entry criteria. One included patients with increased systolic blood pressure and/or increased diastolic blood pressure and any evidence of target organ damage.[84] Another included patients with an elevated diastolic blood pressure and eye changes,[85] while the third included patients with elevated diastolic blood pressure but did not provide any information explicitly on patients with target organ damage.[86] The only statistically significant finding was that patients who received nifedipine achieved their target blood pressure more quickly than those who received nitroprusside.[85]

Table 7.6. Three small Level 2b trials that treated hypertensive emergencies.

Patients	Intervention	Outcomes	Results
SBP over 200 mm Hg and/or DBP over 110 mm Hg and evidence of target organ damage.[84]	Nitroprusside intravenously versus urapidil intravenously	1. BP 185/95 mm Hg at 90 minutes 2. Major adverse effects (hypotension)	1. NNT 12 (NNH 5 to NNT 40) 2. NNH 3 (NNH 3 to NNT 22)
DBP over 130 mm Hg and eye ground changes.[85]	Nitroprusside intravenously versus nifedipine orally	Time at which DBP was 120 mm Hg or lower	14.2 +/−12.6 hours in nitroprusside group versus 4.5 +/−4.5 hours in nifedipine group ($p<0.05$)
DBP over 120 mm Hg and patients with target organ damage not explicitly excluded.[86]	Nifedipine sublingual versus captopril sublingual versus nifedipine sublingual and clonidine intramuscular versus nifedipine sublingual and furosemide intravenously	1. Change in blood pressure 2. Adverse effects	1. No significant differences between blood pressures in any groups 2. Patients who received clonidine complained of a bad taste

SBP   systolic blood pressure
DBP   diastolic blood pressure
NNT   number needed to treat
NNH   number needed to harm

Treatment for hypertensive urgencies

We were unable to identify any high quality studies that addressed the following issues: what blood pressure defines an urgency, how quickly blood pressure should be decreased in a hypertensive urgency, when maintenance therapy should be started or whether patients with hypertensive urgencies should be treated in observed settings. We found ten trials that addressed therapy in patients with hypertensive urgencies (Table 7.7). [87,88](Tx: Llb, L2b) Trials defined hypertensive urgency differently; the most consistently used definition was a diastolic blood pressure of greater than 120 mm Hg. Methodological problems of the trials included small sample size,[88-92] lack of randomization,[93] open label design,[88,93] lack of follow-up,[94] and contamination.[92]

Few studies looked at outcomes more than 24 hours after randomization; follow-up ranged from 15 minutes to one week. Moreover, the trials variously defined the outcome of response to therapy, and none looked at long-term control or important cardiovascular endpoints. Several agents, such as lacidipine, nicardipine, labetalol, and urapidil, clearly decreased short-term blood pressure levels. Nifedipine was noted to cause a stroke in one study.[90] A review article that addressed adverse effects of agents given for hypertensive urgencies and emergencies concluded that short-acting nifedipine should be avoided because of its potential for precipitating both stroke and myocardial infarction.[95]

Table 7.7. A comparison of 10 trials that treated hypertensive urgencies.

Patients	Intervention	Outcomes	Results
DBP over 120 mm Hg[87]	Nicardipine PO 30 mg versus placebo	DBP under 100 mm Hg	NNT 2 (1 to 5)
DBP at 120 mm Hg or higher[89]	Nifedipine PO 20 mg versus nicardipine PO 20 mg versus captopril PO 25 mg	1. DBP at 110 mm Hg or lower	1. Nifedipine versus nicardipine NNT 24 (NNH 5 to NNT 9) nicardipine versus captopril NNT 18 (NNH 4 to NNT 9) nifedipine versus captopril NNT 77 (NNH 5 to NNT 6)
		2. Adverse effects	2. No difference in adverse effects except nifedipine increased heart rate compared with other agents
DBP 110 to 140 mm Hg[96]	Labetalol PO 100 mg versus labetalol PO 200 mg versus labetalol PO 300 mg	DBP at 100 mm Hg or lower or 30 mm Hg reduction in DBP	100 versus 200 mg: NNT 6 (NNH 1 to NNT 4); 100 versus 300 mg: NNT 12 (NNH 2 to NNT 3)
DBP at 120 mm Hg or higher[90]	Lacidipine PO 4 mg versus nifedipine PO 20 mg	1. Decrease in DBP more than 25% of baseline at 8 and 24 hours	1. NNT 2 (1 to 8)
		2. Adverse effects	2. One patient in nifedipine group had a stroke 30 minutes after the dose, blood pressure decreased from 210/125 mm Hg to 120/80 mm Hg

Table 7.7 continued. A comparison of 10 trials that treated hypertensive urgencies.

Patients	Intervention	Outcomes	Results
DBP at 120 mm Hg or higher [97]	Nifedipine PO 20 mg versus clonidine PO 0.1 mg repeated every hour	1. DBP at 100 mm Hg or lower	1. NNT 2 (1 to 2)
		2. Adverse effects	2. Significant increase in heart rate in nifedipine group
DBP 116 to 139 mm Hg [91]	Three different combinations of chlorthalidone and clonidine	Fall in DBP of 20 mm Hg or DBP less than 105 mm Hg	No differences between groups
DBP 100 to 114 mm Hg [92]	Enalapril at 1.25 mg IV every 6 hours versus placebo	DBP less than 95 mm Hg	NNT 4 (NNH 1 to NNT 19)
SBP over 200 mm Hg and/or DBP over 110 mm Hg [93]	Urapidil IV 25 mg, then 12.5 mg if no response versus nifedipine sublingual 10 mg, repeated if no response	SBP less than 180 mm Hg or DBP less than 100 mm Hg	NNT 5 (2 to 55)
SBP 200 to 250 mm Hg or DBP 110 to 140 mm Hg [94]	Nifedipine PO 10 mg versus nitrendipine PO 5 mg	Decrease of 20 mm Hg or more in SBP and 15 mm Hg or more in DBP	NNT 1000 (NNH 7 to NNT 7)
DBP at 120 mm Hg or higher [88]	Nifedipine PO 10 mg repeated two times if necessary versus labetalol PO 200 mg followed by 100 mg or 200 mg at 2 hours if necessary	DBP 110 mm Hg or lower	NNT 6 (NNH 2 to NNT 10)

Our practiced judgments

We treat patients with hypertensive emergencies with intravenous antihypertensive agents in closely observed settings, such as intensive care units. We treat patients with hypertensive urgencies in outpatient settings with close follow-up, ranging from less than three to several days. We use oral agents and avoid short-acting calcium channel blockers. We choose agents based on patients' past histories of response and whether the agents are known to decrease cardiovascular morbidity and mortality. We often use more than one drug to treat patients with urgencies.

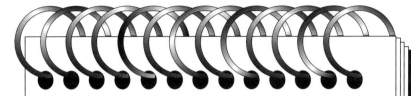

Patient Notes

Mrs Irma Real

- BP 165/98 mm Hg
- Recent shortness of breath

Actions

We obtained an ECG that showed left ventricular hypertrophy but no evidence of ischemia. We also obtained an echocardiogram that showed mild left ventricular systolic dysfunction.

We encouraged her (again) to quit smoking. We added a thiazide diuretic and an ACE inhibitor to her medication regimen. Within two weeks, her shortness of breath improved and her BP was 148/92 mm Hg.

Mr Dan Taylor

- BP 200/114 mm Hg
- Forgot medications for one week

Actions

We immediately restarted his prior three-drug regimen and had him take blood pressure measurements at home. Our nurse practitioner called him the following morning and ascertained that he was feeling well and had no headaches or new symptoms. He reported that his self-monitored blood pressure had decreased within a few hours of restarting his medications. He vowed never to forget his medications again. We saw him back in follow-up one week later; his blood pressure was near control levels.

Summary bottom lines

- Monitor the following parameters during follow-up visits with hypertensive patients:
  - Blood pressure level
  - Adherence to lifestyle and therapeutic recommendations
  - Adverse effects of prescribed therapeutic recommendations
  - Target organ damage that is clinically and physiologically manifested
  - Concomitant cardiovascular risk factors
  - Concomitant, coincident illnesses and therapies
  - Psychosocial circumstances, preferences, and values

- Target treatment blood pressure levels to less than 140 mm Hg systolic and less than 85 to 90 mm Hg diastolic. In diabetics, target lower blood pressure levels to less than 135 to 140 mm Hg systolic and less than 75 to 80 mm Hg. (Level 1 evidence)

- Use selected history-taking, physical examination, and laboratory testing to evaluate target organ damage. (Consensus opinion)

- Consider how the presence of comorbid risk factors and conditions should influence your choice of antihypertensive therapy. (Consensus opinion) For example, if a patient develops coronary artery disease and has previously been prescribed a diuretic for hypertension, consider changing therapy to a beta-blocker for its antianginal effect.

- Review a patient's medications for other conditions, both prescription and over-the-counter, to ensure that they do not interfere with blood pressure. (Consensus opinion)

- Ask about adverse effects of antihypertensive medications, and give patients information about adverse effects. (Consensus opinion) Though side effects are believed to occur in between 10% and 18% of people taking antihypertensive drugs, one survey found 41% of patients reported adverse drug effects and only 31% were satisfied with the amount of information they received about these effects.

- Aim for at least 80% adherence to the therapeutic regimen you prescribe. Patients at this level of compliance are most apt to achieve expected reductions in blood pressure. Recognize that 50% adherence is the norm, with considerable variation from week to week. Look for clues that your patient may be noncompliant. These include uncontrolled blood pressure, loss of responsiveness to a previously adequate dose of treatment, and nonattendance at appointments. Directly ask your patient, "Have you ever missed any of your pills?" (This last statement does have evidence to support its accuracy.) (Consensus opinion)

- Consider interventions to improve medication adherence. Those that have proven successful are automated telephone patient monitoring and counseling, single morning dosing, frequent reinforcement from a medical professional, and rewards for improvements. (Level 1 evidence)

- Educate your patients about hypertension and its management, realizing that there is little evidence showing education improves clinical outcomes. (Consensus opinion)

- Recommended revisit intervals for hypertensive patients whose blood pressure and treatment is stable varies between three months and six months. Various national guidelines also suggest monthly visits after drug therapy is initiated until three blood pressure readings are below the target. Monthly visits also are recommended for patients with symptoms, severe hypertension, intolerance of medications, or target organ damage. In general, physicians lengthen revisit intervals for routine visits, and shorten them when changing management. (Consensus opinion)

- Consider using multidisciplinary care with nurses, pharmacists, nurse-practitioners, and/or physicians' assistants to help ensure adequate follow-up of patients with hypertension. (Consensus opinion)

- Treat hypertensive emergencies with intravenous agents in closely observed settings. Treat hypertensive urgencies with oral medications in outpatient settings, with close and frequent follow-up. Avoid excessive reduction in blood pressure, which can precipitate renal, cerebral or coronary ischemia. (Consensus opinion)

We identified information for this chapter by searching MEDLINE from 1966 to 2000. We searched for English language, human-related literature relevant to the management of hypertension, hypertensive emergencies, and hypertensive urgencies. We specifically looked for trials that addressed the following: target blood pressure levels, timing of titration of medications and follow-up visits, type of follow-up care, patient education, and strategies to improve adherence. We also looked for diagnostic studies that addressed accuracy of detecting target organ damage. We screened approximately 2000 titles and/or abstracts to help identify the highest quality relevant information to include in the chapter.

References

1. Ramsay L, Williams B, Johnston G, *et al.* Guidelines for management of hypertension: report of the third working party of the British Hypertension Society. *J Hum Hypertens* 1999; **13**:569-92.

2. Feldman RD, Campbell N, Larochelle P, *et al.* 1999 Canadian recommendations for the management of hypertension. Task Force for the Development of the 1999 Canadian Recommendations for the Management of Hypertension. *CMAJ* 1999; **161**:S1-17.

3. Joint National Committee on Prevention, Detection, Evaluation, and Treatment of High Blood Pressure. *Report of the Joint National Committee on Prevention, Detection, Evaluation, and Treatment of High Blood Pressure.* 6th ed. Bethesda (MD): National Institutes of Health, National Heart, Lung, and Blood Institute, 1997.

4. Holmen J, Aursnes I, Forsdahl A, *et al.* Report: *NSAM's handling program: hypertension* (Norwegian College of General Practitioner's handling program for general practice). Bergen, Norway: Norwegian College of General Practitioners, 1993.

5. Steven ID, Wing L. Control and cardiovascular risk factors of hypertension. An assessment of a sample of patients. *Aust Fam Physician* 1999; **28**:45-8.

6. Klungel OH, De Boer A, Paes AH, Seidell JC, Nagelkerke NJ, Bakker A. Undertreatment of hypertension in a population-based study in The Netherlands. *J Hypertens* 1998; **16**:1371-8.

7. Mulrow PJ. Detection and control of hypertension in the population: the United States experience. *Am J Hypertens* 1998; **11**:744-6.

8. Joffres MR, Ghadirian P, Fodor JG, Petrasovits A, Chockalingam A, Hamet P. Awareness, treatment, and control of hypertension in Canada. *Am J Hypertens* 1997; **10**:1097-102.

9. McAlister FA, Teo KK, Lewanczuk RZ, Wells G, Montague TJ. Contemporary practice patterns in the management of newly diagnosed hypertension. *CMAJ* 1997; **157**:23-30.

10. Adults taking action to control their blood pressure — United States, 1990. *MMWR* 1994; **43**:509-11.

11. Foss FA, Dickinson E, Hills M, Thomson A, Wilson V, Ebrahim S. Missed opportunities for the prevention of cardiovascular disease among British hypertensives in primary care. *Br J Gen Pract* 1996; **46**:571-5.

12. Stewart IM. Relation of reduction in pressure to first myocardial infarction in patients receiving treatment for severe hypertension. *Lancet* 1979; **i**:861-5.

13. Farnett L, Mulrow CD, Linn WD, Lucey CR, Tuley MR. The J-curve phenomenon and the treatment of hypertension. Is there a point beyond which pressure reduction is dangerous? *JAMA* 1991; **265**:489-95.

14. McAlister FA. Using evidence to resolve clinical controversies: is aggressive antihypertensive therapy harmful? *Evidence-Based Med* 1999; **4**:4-6.

15. Hannson L. The BBB Study: the effect of intensified antihypertensive treatment on the level of blood pressure, side-effects, morbidity and mortality in "well-treated" hypertensive patients. Behandla Blodtryck Battre. *Blood Press* 1994; **3**:248-54.

16. Hansson L, Zanchetti A, Carruthers SG, *et al.* Effects of intensive blood-pressure lowering and low-dose aspirin in patients with hypertension: principal results of the Hypertension Optimal Treatment (HOT) randomised trial. HOT Study Group. *Lancet* 1998; **351**:1755-62.

17. UK Prospective Diabetes Study Group. Tight blood pressure control and risk of macrovascular and microvascular complications in type 2 diabetes: UKPDS 38 [published erratum appears in *BMJ* 1999; **318**:29]. *BMJ* 1998; **317**:703-13.

18. Merlo J, Ranstam J, Liedholm H, *et al.* Incidence of myocardial infarction in elderly men being treated with antihypertensive drugs: population based cohort study. *BMJ* 1996; **313**:457-61.

19. Cooper SP, Hardy RJ, Labarthe DR, *et al*. The relation between degree of blood pressure reduction and mortality among hypertensives in the Hypertension Detection and Follow-Up Program. *Am J Epidemiol* 1988; **127**:387-403.

20. McAlister FA, Straus SE, Sackett DL. Why we need large, simple studies of the clinical examination: the problem and a proposed solution. CARE-COAD1 group. Clinical Assessment of the Reliability of the Examination-Chronic Obstructive Airways Disease Group [published erratum appears in *Lancet* 2000; **355**:580]. *Lancet* 1999; **354**:1721-4.

21. World Health Organization-International Society of Hypertension. Guidelines Subcommittee. 1999 World Health Organization-International Society of Hypertension Guidelines for the Management of Hypertension. Guidelines Subcommittee. *J Hypertens* 1999; **17**:151-83.

22. Gifford RW Jr, Kirkendall W, O'Connor DT, Weidman W. Office evaluation of hypertension. A statement for health professionals by a writing group of the Council for High Blood Pressure Research, American Heart Association. *Circulation* 1989; **79**:721-31.

23. Joint National Committee on Prevention, Detection, Evaluation, and Treatment of High Blood Pressure. The sixth report of the Joint National Committee on Prevention, Detection, Evaluation, and Treatment of High Blood Pressure [published erratum appears in *Arch Intern Med* 1998; **158**:573]. *Arch Intern Med* 1997; **157**:2413-46.

24. Badgett RG, Lucey CR, Mulrow CD. Can the clinical examination diagnose left-sided heart failure in adults? *JAMA* 1997; **277**:1712-19.

25. Cook DJ, Simel DL. The Rational Clinical Examination. Does this patient have abnormal central venous pressure? *JAMA* 1996; **275**:630-4.

26. Etchells E, Bell C, Robb K. Does this patient have an abnormal systolic murmur? *JAMA* 1997; **277**:564-71.

27. Yu T, Mitchell P, Berry G, Li W, Wang JJ. Retinopathy in older persons without diabetes and its relationship to hypertension. *Arch Ophthalmol* 1998; **116**:83-9.

28. Keith NM, Wagener HP, Barker NW. Some different types of essential hypertension: their course and prognosis. *Am J Med Sci* 1974; **268**:336-45.

29. Khagan A, Aurell E, Dobree J. A note on signs in the fundus occulae in arterial hypertension: conventional assessment and significance. *Bull World Health Organ* 1966; **34**:955-60.

30. Post WS, Larson MG, Levy D. Impact of left ventricular structure on the incidence of hypertension. The Framingham Heart Study. *Circulation* 1994; **90**:179-85.

31. Curb JD, Borhani NO, Blaszkowski TP, Zimbaldi N, Fotiu S, Williams W. Patient-perceived side effects to antihypertensive drugs. *Am J Prev Med* 1985; **1**:36-40.

32. Morris LA. A survey of patients' receipt of prescription drug information. *Med Care* 1982; **20**:596-605.

33. Enlund H, Vainio K, Wallenius S, Poston JW. Adverse drug effects and the need for drug information. *Med Care* 1991; **29**:558-64.

34. Anderson RB, Hollenberg NK, Williams GH. Physical Symptoms Distress Index: a sensitive tool to evaluate the impact of pharmacological agents on quality of life. *Arch Intern Med* 1999; **159**:693-700.

35. Black DM, Brand RJ, Greenlick M, Hughes G, Smith J. Compliance to treatment for hypertension in elderly patients: the SHEP pilot study. Systolic Hypertension in the Elderly Program. *J Gerontol* 1987; **42**:552-7.

36. Maronde RF, Chan LS, Larsen FJ, Strandberg LR, Laventurier MF, Sullivan SR. Underutilization of antihypertensive drugs and associated hospitalization. *Med Care* 1989; **27**:1159-66.

37. Caro JJ, Speckman JL. Existing treatment strategies: does noncompliance make a difference? *J Hypertens* (Suppl) 1998; **16**:S31-4.

38. Jones JK, Gorkin L, Lian JF, Staffa JA, Fletcher AP. Discontinuation of and changes in treatment after start of new courses of antihypertensive drugs: a study of a United Kingdom population. *BMJ* 1995; **311**:293-5.

39. Bailey JE, Lee MD, Somes GW, Graham RL. Risk factors for antihypertensive medication refill failure by patients under Medicaid managed care. *Clin Ther* 1996; **18**:1252-62.

40. Kyngas H, Lahdenpera T. Compliance of patients with hypertension and associated factors. *J Adv Nurs* 1999; **29**:832-9.

41. Kravitz RL, Hays RD, Sherbourne CD, *et al*. Recall of recommendations and adherence to advice among patients with chronic medical conditions. *Arch Intern Med* 1993; **153**:1869-78.

42. Haynes RB, Taylor DW, Sackett DL, Gibson ES, Bernholz CD, Mukherjee J. Can simple clinical measurements detect patient noncompliance? *Hypertension* 1980; **2**:757-64.

43. Stephenson BJ, Rowe BH, Haynes RB, Macharia WM, Leon G. Is this patient taking the treatment as prescribed? *JAMA* 1993; **269**:2779-81.

44. Balazovjech I, Hnilica P Jr. Compliance with antihypertensive treatment in consultation rooms for hypertensive patients. *J Hum Hypertens* 1993; **7**:581-3.

45. Heurtin-Roberts S, Reisin E. The relation of culturally influenced lay models of hypertension to compliance with treatment. *Am J Hypertens* 1992; **5**:787-92.

46. Sharkness CM, Snow DA. The patient's view of hypertension and compliance. *Am J Prev Med* 1992; **8**:141-6.

47. Dusing R, Weisser B, Mengden T, Vetter H. Changes in antihypertensive therapy — the role of adverse effects and compliance. *Blood Press* 1998; **7**:313-15.

48. Caro JJ, Salas M, Speckman JL, Raggio G, Jackson JD. Persistence with treatment for hypertension in actual practice. *CMAJ* 1999; **160**:31-7.

49. Caro JJ, Speckman JL, Salas M, Raggio G, Jackson JD. Effect of initial drug choice on persistence with antihypertensive therapy: the importance of actual practice data. *CMAJ* 1999; **160**:41-6.

50. Rizzo JA, Simons WR. Variations in compliance among hypertensive patients by drug class: implications for health care costs. *Clin Ther* 1997; **19**:1446-57.

51. Monane M, Bohn RL, Gurwitz JH, Glynn RJ, Levin R, Avorn J. The effects of initial drug choice and comorbidity on antihypertensive therapy compliance: results from a population-based study in the elderly. *Am J Hypertens* 1997; **10**:697-704.

52. Gilbert JR, Evans CE, Haynes RB, Tugwell P. Predicting compliance with a regimen of digoxin therapy in family practice. *CMAJ* 1980; **123**:119-22.

53. Guerrero D, Rudd P, Bryant-Kosling C, Middleton B, Middleton BF. Antihypertensive medication-taking. Investigation of a simple regimen [published erratum appears in *Am J Hypertens* 1993; **6**:982]. *Am J Hypertens* 1993; **6**:586-92.

54. Lee JY, Kusek JW, Greene PG, *et al*. Assessing medication adherence by pill count and electronic monitoring in the African American Study of Kidney Disease and Hypertension (AASK) Pilot Study. *Am J Hypertens* 1996; **9**:719-25.

55. Mallion JM, Meilhac B, Tremel F, Calvez R, Bertholom N. Use of a microprocessor-equipped tablet box in monitoring compliance with antihypertensive treatment. *J Cardiovasc Pharmacol* 1992; **19**:S41-8.

56. Christensen DB, Williams B, Goldberg HI, Martin DP, Engelberg R, LoGerfo JP. Assessing compliance to antihypertensive medications using computer-based pharmacy records. *Med Care* 1997; **35**:1164-70.

57. Cronin CC, Higgins TM, Murphy MB, Ferriss JB. Supervised drug administration in patients with refractory hypertension unmasking noncompliance. *Postgrad Med J* 1997; **73**:239-40.

58. Haynes RB, Montague P, Oliver T, McKibbon KA, Brouwers MC, Kanani R. Interventions for helping patients to follow prescriptions for medications. (Cochrane Review) In: *The Cochrane Library, Issue 2*, 2000. Oxford: Update Software.

59. Friedman RH, Kazis LE, Jette A, *et al*. A telecommunications system for monitoring and counseling patients with hypertension. Impact on medication adherence and blood pressure control. *Am J Hypertens* 1996; **9**:285-92.

60. Logan AG, Milne BJ, Achber C, Campbell WP, Haynes RB. Work-site treatment of hypertension by specially trained nurses. A controlled trial. *Lancet* 1979; **ii**:1175-8.

61. Baird MG, Bentley-Taylor MM, Carruthers SG, *et al.* A study of efficacy, tolerance and compliance of once-daily versus twice-daily metoprolol (Betaloc) in hypertension. Betaloc Compliance Canadian Cooperative Study Group. *Clin Invest Med* 1984; **7**:95-102.

62. Becker LA, Glanz K, Sobel E, Mossey J, Zinn SL, Knott KA. A randomized trial of special packaging of antihypertensive medications. *J Fam Pract* 1986; **22**:357-61.

63. Johnson AL, Taylor DW, Sackett DL, Dunnett CW, Shimizu AG. Self-recording of blood pressure in the management of hypertension. *CMAJ* 1978; **119**:1034-9.

64. Haynes RB, Sackett DL, Gibson ES, *et al.* Improvement of medication compliance in uncontrolled hypertension. *Lancet* 1976; **i**:1265-8.

65. Sackett DL, Haynes RB, Gibson ES, *et al.* Randomised clinical trial of strategies for improving medication compliance in primary hypertension. *Lancet* 1975; **i**:1205-7.

66. Roca-Cusachs A, Sort D, Altimira J, *et al.* The impact of a patient education programme in the control of hypertension. *J Hum Hypertens* 1991; **5**:437-41.

67. Devine EC, Reifschneider E. A meta-analysis of the effects of psychoeducational care in adults with hypertension. *Nurs Res* 1995; **44**:237-45.

68. Krishna S, Balas EA, Spencer DC, Griffin JZ, Boren SA. Clinical trials of interactive computerized patient education: implications for family practice. *J Fam Pract* 1997; **45**:25-33.

69. Said MB, Consoli S, Jean J. Comparative study between a computer-aided education and habitual education techniques for hypertensive patients. *J Am Med Inform Assoc* 1994; **1**:10-14.

70. Ribacke M. Treatment preferences, return visit planning and factors affecting hypertension practice amongst general practitioners and internal medicine specialists (the General Practitioner Hypertension Practice Study). *J Intern Med* 1995; **237**:473-8.

71. Lichtenstein MJ, Steele MA, Hoehn TP, Bulpitt CJ, Coles EC. Visit frequency for essential hypertension: observed associations. *J Fam Pract* 1989; **28**:667-72.

72. Tobacman JK, Zeitler RR, Cilursu AM, Mori M. Variation in physician opinion about scheduling of return visits for common ambulatory care conditions. *J Gen Intern Med* 1992; **7**:312-16.

73. Schwartz LM, Woloshin S, Wasson JH, Renfrew RA, Welch HG. Setting the revisit interval in primary care. *J Gen Intern Med* 1999; **14**:230-5.

74. Flack JM, Yunis C, Preisser J, *et al.* The rapidity of drug dose escalation influences blood pressure response and adverse effects burden in patients with hypertension: the Quinapril Titration Interval Management Evaluation (ATIME) Study. ATIME Research Group. *Arch Intern Med* 2000; **160**:1842-7.

75. Zarnke KB, Feagan BG, Mahon JL, Feldman RD. A randomized study comparing a patient-directed hypertension management strategy with usual office-based care. *Am J Hypertens* 1997; **10**:58-67.

76. Strate M, Vaeth M, Harvald B. Twenty-one-year survival of primary hypertensive patients allocated to care in general practice or in specialized hypertension clinic. An observational study of 831 hypertensive patients. *Blood Press* 1997; **6**:88-95.

77. McInnes GT, McGhee SM. Delivery of care for hypertension. *J Hum Hypertens* 1995; **9**:429-33.

78. Woollard J, Beilin L, Lord T, Puddey I, MacAdam D, Rouse I. A controlled trial of nurse counselling on lifestyle change for hypertensives treated in general practice: preliminary results. *Clin Exp Pharmacol Physiol* 1995; **22**:466-8.

79. Bero LA, Mays NB, Barjesteh K, Bond C. Expanding the roles of outpatient pharmacists: effects on health services utilisation, costs, and patient outcomes. (Cochrane Review) In: *The Cochrane Library, Issue 2*, 2000. Oxford: Update Software.

80. Hawkins DW, Fiedler FP, Douglas HL, Eschbach RC. Evaluation of a clinical pharmacist in caring for hypertensive and diabetic patients. *Am J Hosp Pharm* 1979; **36**:1321-5.

81. McKenney JM, Slining JM, Henderson HR, Devins D, Barr M. The effect of clinical pharmacy services on patients with essential hypertension. *Circulation* 1973; **48**:1104-11.

82. Bogden PE, Abbott RD, Williamson P, Onopa JK, Koontz LM. Comparing standard care with a physician and pharmacist team approach for uncontrolled hypertension. *J Gen Intern Med* 1998; **13**:740-5.

83. Kitiyakara C, Guzman NJ. Malignant hypertension and hypertensive emergencies. *J Am Soc Nephrol* 1998; **9**:133-42.

84. Hirschl MM, Binder M, Bur A, *et al.* Safety and efficacy of urapidil and sodium nitroprusside in the treatment of hypertensive emergencies. *Intensive Care Med* 1997; **23**:885-8.

85. Franklin C, Nightingale S, Mamdani B. A randomized comparison of nifedipine and sodium nitroprusside in severe hypertension. *Chest* 1986; **90**:500-3.

86. Pascale C, Zampaglione B, Marchisio M. Management of hypertensive crisis: nifedipine in comparison with captopril, clonidine and furosemide. *Curr Ther Res Clin Exp* 1992; **51**:9-18.

87. Habib GB, Dunbar LM, Rodrigues R, Neale AC, Friday KJ. Evaluation of the efficacy and safety of oral nicardipine in treatment of urgent hypertension: a multicenter, randomized, double-blind, parallel, placebo-controlled clinical trial. *Am Heart J* 1995; **129**:917-23.

88. McDonald AJ, Yealy DM, Jacobson S. Oral labetalol versus oral nifedipine in hypertensive urgencies in the ED. *Am J Emerg Med* 1993; **11**:460-3.

89. Komsuoglu B, Sengun B, Bayram A, Komsuoglu SS. Treatment of hypertensive urgencies with oral nifedipine, nicardipine, and captopril. *Angiology* 1991; **42**:447-54.

90. Sanchez M, Sobrino J, Ribera L, Adrian MJ, Torres M, Coca A. Long-acting lacidipine versus short-acting nifedipine in the treatment of asymptomatic acute blood pressure increase. *J Cardiovasc Pharmacol* 1999; **33**:479-84.

91. Zeller KR, Von Kuhnert L, Matthews C. Rapid reduction of severe asymptomatic hypertension. A prospective, controlled trial. *Arch Intern Med* 1989; **149**:2186-9.

92. Rutledge J, Ayers C, Davidson R, *et al.* Effect of intravenous enalaprilat in moderate and severe systemic hypertension. *Am J Cardiol* 1988; **62**:1062-7.

93. Hirschl MM, Seidler D, Zeiner A, *et al.* Intravenous urapidil versus sublingual nifedipine in the treatment of hypertensive urgencies. *Am J Emerg Med* 1993; **11**:653-6.

94. Rohr G, Reimnitz P, Blanke P. Treatment of hypertensive emergency. Comparison of a new dosage form of the calcium antagonist nitrendipine with nifedipine capsules. *Intensive Care Med* 1994; **20**:268-71.

95. Grossman E, Messerli FH, Grodzicki T, Kowey P. Should a moratorium be placed on sublingual nifedipine capsules given for hypertensive emergencies and pseudoemergencies? *JAMA* 1996; **276**:1328-31.

96. Gonzalez ER, Peterson MA, Racht EM, Ornato JP, Due DL. Dose-response evaluation of oral labetalol in patients presenting to the emergency department with accelerated hypertension. *Ann Emerg Med* 1991; **20**:333-8.

97. Jaker M, Atkin S, Soto M, Schmid G, Brosch F. Oral nifedipine vs oral clonidine in the treatment of urgent hypertension. *Arch Intern Med* 1989; **149**:260-5.

CHAPTER 8

What do we do if our patient's blood pressure is "difficult-to-control"?

Jane E O'Rorke
W Scott Richardson

What do we mean by "difficult-to-control" blood pressure?

What can cause blood pressure to be "difficult-to-control," and how frequent are these causes?

How can we evaluate individual patients with "difficult-to-control" blood pressure to determine the cause(s) and adjust our plans?

Summary bottom lines

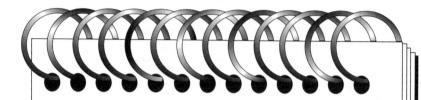

Patient Notes

Mrs Ova Whelms, age 49, homemaker

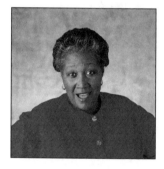

- Uncontrolled hypertension
- Father had hypertension and died of a stroke at age 42
- Prescribed a thiazide, a beta-blocker, an ACE inhibitor, and an alpha-1 antagonist

Reason for visit

- Follow-up for her hypertension

Clinical findings

- BP 218/126 mm Hg
- Obese BMI 28
- No symptoms or findings suggestive of target organ damage

Clinical question

How do we differentiate among the causes of "resistant" hypertension in adult patients?

What do we mean by "difficult-to-control" blood pressure?

We could not find a universally accepted definition of blood pressure that is "difficult-to-control," "uncontrolled," "resistant," or "refractory." One consensus-based national guideline from the United States defines resistant hypertension as blood pressure that cannot be reduced to below 140/90 mm Hg (or below 160 mm Hg for isolated systolic hypertension) in patients who are adhering to adequate and appropriately dosed triple drug regimens.[1] While we may use this definition for many patients, for some we would aim for even lower blood pressure targets and consider them "difficult-to-control" if these could not be reached.

Both clinical experience and research surveys suggest that "difficult-to-control" blood pressure is common in everyday practice. For example, population and clinic surveys in North America, Europe, and Australia show that as many as 50% to 75% of people with diagnosed hypertension do not meet target blood pressure levels.[2] One recent large trial involving 19 196 patients found that as many as 50% of the eligible enrollees had uncontrolled blood pressure levels at baseline despite already receiving antihypertensive therapy. Of these "uncontrolled" hypertensive patients, 59% were receiving one-drug regimens and 41% were receiving two-drug regimens. During the course of the trial, which targeted diastolic blood pressures levels as low as 80 mm Hg, 72% of the patients required multiple-drug regimens.[3] A second large trial in hypertensive diabetic people found that 60% of the participants required two or more drugs to achieve target blood pressure levels of less than 150/85 mm Hg. A third of the participants required three or more drugs.[4] These findings confirm that even in settings with close follow-up, blood pressure control can be difficult to achieve.

What can cause blood pressure to be "difficult-to-control," and how frequent are these causes?

To make the list of causes of resistant hypertension more manageable, we have grouped them into eight categories (Box 8.1). As you review this list, consider that an individual patient may have more than one factor causing resistance to treatment.

Box 8.1. Categories of causes of "difficult-to-control" blood pressure.

- Inaccurate blood pressure measurement
- White-coat hypertension
- Disease progression
- Suboptimal treatments
- Nonadherence to prescribed treatments
- Antagonizing substances
- Coexisting conditions
- Secondary hypertension

We have found relatively little evidence regarding the frequency with which these eight categories are found to be the explanations for "difficult-to-control" blood pressure. A small descriptive survey from a referral clinic reported the following frequencies: suboptimal treatment, 40%; nonadherence to prescribed therapy, 10% to 50%; white-coat hypertension, 2% to 4%; and secondary causes, 10%.[5] We reckon the relative proportions of these explanations could be quite different in primary care settings, with lower rates of secondary causes, but we have relatively little direct evidence. We address each category below.

Inaccurate blood pressure measurement

As discussed in Chapter 2, the results of blood pressure measurement can depend on using proper technique and the conditions under which the measurements are made. Before concluding that a patient has resistant hypertension that requires detailed testing and escalating treatments, we repeat blood pressure measurements under good conditions and with technique as close to ideal as possible. See Chapter 2 for recommendations on good technique and examining conditions.

White-coat hypertension

As also discussed in Chapter 2, some patients have acceptably controlled blood pressure when outside the doctor's office, yet have higher readings when examined by the clinician. Earlier we discussed how this event could distort our conclusions about whether such patients even have high blood pressure. In the present context, we can see how this same phenomenon might lead us to believe incorrectly that a patient's blood pressure was poorly controlled. As discussed more in Chapter 2, we can examine this possible contributor by enlisting the aid of others to measure the patient's blood pressure multiple times elsewhere. Example methods include visits to nurses or other health care workers, self-monitoring with home sphygmomanometers, or ambulatory blood pressure monitoring. If good technique is used with well-calibrated equipment, these other measurements can be integrated with those in the doctor's office to create a fuller picture of blood pressure control. If all the readings were persistently elevated, we would conclude that the blood pressure had not yet reached target values.

Disease progression

With time, adults with hypertension will gradually develop further increases in recorded blood pressure.[6] Such increases occur with both treated and untreated patients, although presumably more quickly with the latter. Potential contributors include the stiffening of arterial walls with age-related declines in vessel resilience, advancing atherosclerosis, increasing renal insufficiency, and the steady accumulation of coexisting conditions that may worsen blood pressure. We found no recent, rigorous evidence about the relative frequencies of these contributing factors or about how frequently resistant hypertension is explained only by disease progression. Without such evidence to guide us, we seldom conclude that "difficult-to-control" blood pressure represents solely disease progression until we have excluded other causes.

Suboptimal treatments

For any number of reasons, patients may not be prescribed optimal, individualized programs of antihypertensive treatment. As mentioned, many patients require aggressive treatment with multiple-drug regimens to achieve target blood pressure levels. We found that a survey of American physicians showed as many as 25% to 33% self-reported that they did not intensify antihypertensive regimens in people who were not at nationally suggested target levels.[7] They self-reported less intensive blood pressure lowering practices for systolic pressures and in older patients.[7] Reasons underlying physicians' lack of aggressiveness in treatment were not clear.

Another population-based survey from the United States showed certain groups of people with particular characteristics were more likely to have suboptimal control of their hypertension than others.[8] The group with the highest systolic blood pressure included young men with little professed knowledge of hypertension and little credence that not taking their medication was a threat to their health. Such people were the most likely not to take antihypertensive medications and to have changed or discontinued medication without consulting a clinician.

To detect suboptimal treatment, we can review patients' complete medication list, dietary habits, exercise pattern, and any other adjuncts being used. For each drug prescribed, we can ask whether its dose, route and frequency conforms with both what we know about its rational prescribing and what we know of our patients' unique health status and preferences. Expert opinion suggests that increased dietary sodium that causes hypervolemia frequently plays a large role in resistant hypertension, leading to recommendations for better use of diuretics when patients have "difficult-to-control" blood pressure.[9-11] We found no rigorous evidence about the relative frequency of this or other forms of suboptimal treatment. Even if it were infrequent, since this category is one of the few causes over which we can exert some control, we tend to emphasize frequent reviews of our patients' regimens, to see if their plans are fully optimized. When reviewing an individual patient's regimen, we use the information in Chapters 4, 5, and 6 to guide our adjustments.

Nonadherence

As discussed in Chapter 7, no matter what treatments are prescribed, they cannot help (or harm) patients if they are not taken. For any number of reasons, patients may not be taking medications as prescribed or at all. Of the available methods to ascertain adherence, direct and nonjudgmental questioning of patients is the most feasible in the context of ongoing clinic visits. A systematic review of the discriminatory power of such simple questioning for detecting nonadherence estimated that the sensitivity of the questioning was 55% and the specificity, 87%.[12] (Dx: L2a) See Chapter 7 for recommendations on detecting and managing nonadherence.

Antagonizing substances

Patients may be exposed to any number of prescription and nonprescription drugs and dietary and other substances that can increase blood pressure or counteract the effects of antihypertensive drugs (Box 8.2). We found no or few rigorous studies that evaluated the frequency or magnitude of effects that such substances have on blood pressure.

On this list, the nonsteroidal antiinflammatory drugs (NSAIDs) deserve particular mention. These drugs are among the most commonly prescribed medications, accounting for 5% to 10% of all prescriptions in developed countries.[13, 14] Older patients have a relatively high burden of painful, musculoskeletal conditions for which they are prescribed NSAIDs, while at the same time they have relatively high prevalence of hypertension requiring drug therapy. If NSAIDs raise blood pressure or counteract the effects of antihypertensive drugs, by the sheer force of numbers these agents could have an enormous impact on global blood pressure control.

Box 8.2. Antagonizing substances that may increase blood pressure.

- Adrenal steroids (especially mineralocorticoids)
- Alcohol
- Amphetamines, e.g., appetite suppressants
- Anesthetics, both local and general
- Antidiuretic hormone and angiotensin
- Caffeine
- Cocaine
- Cyclosporine
- Disulfram
- Erythropoietin
- Licorice or carbenoxolone
- MAO inhibitor drugs, combined with tyramine-containing foods or with amphetamine
- Nonsteroidal antiinflammatory drugs (NSAIDs)
- Oral contraceptives
- Sodium-containing medications, e.g., antacids or parenteral antibiotics
- Sympathomimetic agents, e.g., nasal decongestants or bronchodilators
- Withdrawal from agents, e.g., beta-blockers or clonidine

We found two systematic reviews that examined the direction and magnitude of effect that NSAIDs have on blood pressure. One summary of findings from 54 trials found that NSAID therapy increased the mean arterial blood pressure by 1.1 mm Hg in normotensive patients and by 3.3 mm Hg in patients with hypertension.[15](Tx:LIa) Most of these trials were of short duration (less than six weeks), and none included elderly patients. Among NSAID agents, indomethacin had the largest effect on blood pressure, while aspirin had the least. Another systematic review summarized 50 trials and estimated that NSAIDs increased supine mean blood pressure by 5 mm Hg.[16](Tx: LIa)

Coexisting conditions

While usually not considered as causes of secondary hypertension, these disorders may coexist in patients with hypertension and either aggravate blood pressure control or interfere with its treatment (Box 8.3).

Box 8.3. Coexisting conditions that may aggravate blood pressure control.

- Alcohol use, more than 1 to 2 ounces per day
- Anxiety disorders, including hyperventilation or panic attacks
- Delirium, with agitation and autonomic excess
- Hyperinsulinism with insulin resistance
- Obesity
- Pain, both acute and chronic
- Pregnancy
- Sleep apnea
- Smoking

Both clinical experience and research surveys suggest that some of these conditions frequently coexist with hypertension. For example, population surveys have repeatedly shown that as many as 40% of people with hypertension may have coexisting obesity.[17] Obesity can interfere with accurate blood pressure measurement, may predispose to higher true blood pressure, and may interfere with the effectiveness of antihypertensive drugs. Recognizing the co-occurrence of such disorders offers the possibility that treating them could improve blood pressure control, although the extent to which this is true may not be fully known (please see Chapter 6 for more on how comorbid conditions should influence our choice of treatments). The list in Box 8.3 can be used to guide more detailed history, selective examination, chart review or testing in patients with resistant hypertension.

Secondary hypertension

By definition, patients with secondary hypertension have underlying disorders believed to directly cause the high blood pressure. Finding these disorders offers the prospect that patients could receive curative, cause-specific therapy that would result in normalized blood pressure without the need for drug treatments for blood pressure *per se*. We have listed many of the causes in Box 8.4.

Box 8.4. Disorders of secondary hypertension.

Renovascular disorders

- Atherosclerotic renal artery stenosis
- Fibromuscular dysplasia, atheroembolism
- Cholesterol crystal embolism
- Extravascular compression (from tumors, cysts, scarring, etc.)
- Middle aortic syndrome
- Ehlers-Danlos syndrome
- Turner syndrome
- Neurofibromatosis

Renal parenchymal disorders

Acute or chronic renal failure from many disorders, including:

- Glomerulonephritis
- Interstitial nephritis
- Diabetic renal disease
- Connective tissue disorders
- Vasculitides
- Polycystic kidney
- Amyloidosis
- Tuberculosis
- Renal trauma
- Hydronephrosis
- Reflux nephropathy
- Heavy metal poisoning (lead and cadmium)

Renin-secreting tumors

- Cancers of lung, pancreas, kidneys and Wilms' tumor
- Benign tumors of ovaries and hemangiopericytomas

Adrenal disorders

- Cushing's syndrome
- Primary aldosteronism
- Congenital adrenal hyperplasia
- Inborn errors of metabolism (e.g., Liddle's syndrome)
- Pheochromocytoma
- Adrenal adenomas
- Adrenal carcinomas

Other glandular conditions

- Hyperthyroidism
- Hypothyroidism
- Acromegaly
- Hyperparathyroidism

Vascular diseases

- Aortic coarctation

Elevated cardiac output

- Aortic valvular regurgitation
- Paget's disease of bone
- Beriberi
- Arteriovenous fistula (e.g., patent ductus)
- Thyrotoxicosis
- Anemia
- Hyperkinetic circulation

Spinal or peripheral neurologic diseases

- Lesions of upper cord
- Guillain-Barre syndrome
- Lesions of nerves to carotid sinuses
- Autonomic neuropathies
- Acute porphyria
- Peripheral neuropathies

When evaluating patients with resistant hypertension and considering diseases of secondary hypertension, three questions arise: How common are these disorders, either individually or in aggregate? When and in whom should these disorders be considered? How should these disorders be pursued diagnostically? The following three sections address these questions.

How common are these disorders?

We found the frequency of secondary hypertension in primary care settings is uncertain but is probably low among all comers with high blood pressure. We found some evidence addressing the frequency of various secondary causes, but we could not rate the evidence using the levels of evidence scheme. The studies had several potentials for bias and limited generalizability, including selection of patients from referral centers or trial settings.[18-22] They used differing diagnostic criteria, carried out varying diagnostic evaluations, and had varying degrees of follow-up. And as time passes, testing strategies and treatments change, such that patients who were studied in the 1960s through 1980s may no longer be sufficiently similar to patients seen in primary care in the new millennium.

For example, we found a study from a referral clinic in the 1960s that reported the prevalence of renovascular disease was 4.4%, pheochromocytoma, 0.2%, and hyperaldosteronism, 0.4%.[18] At another referral clinic in the early 1970s, the prevalence of renovascular disease was 0.18%, while pheochromocytoma was 0.04%, and hyperaldosteronism was 0.01.[19] Such frequencies obtained at referral centers may be much higher than those seen in modern primary care settings. Regardless, given the state of the evidence, we tentatively reckon that renovascular and renal parenchymal causes of secondary hypertension would be the most common found in primary care practice.

When and in whom should these disorders be considered?

The overall low frequency of disorders of secondary hypertension presents a diagnostic challenge. If we were to search for these diseases in all patients with hypertension, we would find few cases yet expose many of our patients to needless and potentially harmful testing, to say nothing of wasting resources. On the other hand, to never search for them would mean missing diagnoses that could lead to potentially curative therapy and obviate the need for lifelong antihypertensive treatment. This has led experts to recommend selecting patients for further testing who appear to be at higher than average risk for such disorders, based either on epidemiologic issues such as age and gender, or on the presence of certain illness features associated with specific disorders.

For instance, when considering whether to search for renal artery stenosis, experts have recommended selecting patients who present with one or more of the illness patterns listed in Box 8.5.[23]

Box 8.5. Clinical patterns suggestive of renal artery stenosis.

* Severe high blood pressure, particularly with retinal hemorrhages, papilledema, or azotemia
* An acute rise in blood pressure over a previously stable baseline
* Proven age of onset less than 20 years old or older than 50
* An acute elevation of plasma creatinine concentration, either unexplained or after starting treatment
* Moderate or severe high blood pressure in a patient with diffuse atherosclerosis
* Presence of an abdominal bruit
* Resistant hypertension in a patient without a family history of hypertension
* Elevated blood pressure with episodes of recurrent, "flash" pulmonary edema

---

We could not find evidence that addressed how frequently these presenting patterns occurred among all comers with high blood pressure in primary care settings. Furthermore, we found relatively little evidence about how powerfully these features discriminate between those who do and do not have renovascular disease (and indeed, very little about how well any clinical features can detect all the other causes of secondary hypertension). We did find a systematic review of the diagnostic power of abdominal bruits for renal artery stenosis.[24](Dx: L2a) There were only three studies of sufficient rigor to provide credible estimates of accuracy, with sensitivity ranging from 39% to 78% and specificity ranging from 64% to 99%. Thus, for this one finding, the available evidence suggests that it is useful when it is present, but its absence cannot fully exclude renal artery stenosis. Until better evidence becomes available, it may be sensible to use the above selection criteria to select patients in whom to consider further testing for renal artery stenosis.

An alternative approach would be to use a clinical decision or prediction rule to estimate the chance of a disorder causing secondary hypertension in a given patient. For instance, in a study of 477 patients with resistant hypertension or treatment-related azotemia, investigators found several clinical features could be combined to create a summary score that predicted renal artery stenosis with a sensitivity of 72% and a specificity of 90%.[25] If validated in other patient groups by other investigators, this decision rule may help clinicians better predict the presence of renal artery stenosis.

Thus, for renal artery stenosis, some evidence is available to guide our selection of patients in whom to consider further testing. But for many other disorders of secondary hypertension, the evidence is scant or nonexistent. For instance, pheochromocytoma is usually described as causing a clinical pattern of paroxysmal hypertension with headache, palpitations, and diaphoresis. We did not find evidence about how accurately this cluster of findings predicts pheochromocytoma. We did find a well-conducted study of the causes of palpitations seen in one urban medical center; of the 190 patients examined, none had pheochromocytoma.[26] Given the many other causes that were found for palpitations, this evidence suggests that palpitations are not very specific for pheochromocytoma, and, thus, may have limited diagnostic usefulness for this disorder.

How should these disorders be pursued diagnostically?

A full discussion of the testing options for confirming or excluding each cause of secondary hypertension is beyond the scope of this chapter; interested readers should consult other sources.[23, 27] In general, experts have recommended starting with noninvasive and sensitive tests to exclude causes of secondary hypertension safely if the results are negative. Patients with positive results can be considered for more definitive testing. For example, in renal artery stenosis, experts recommend initial testing with either captopril renal scanning or duplex ultrasonography of the renal arteries, followed by renal arteriography if these tests are positive.[27]

How can we evaluate individual patients with "difficult-to-control" blood pressure to determine the cause(s) and adjust our plans?

Ideally, we would like to be able to recommend a coherent strategy for evaluating and managing patients' "difficult-to-control" blood pressure, comprising individually well-studied elements that have been aggregated into a systematic approach that has itself been shown to do more good than harm. We imagine that such a strategy would be powerful enough to find and correct the causes for most cases of resistance, flexible enough to fit patients in different circumstances, efficient enough to be affordable in most health systems, and pragmatic enough to be feasible in most practice settings. Unfortunately, we found little or no evidence beyond expert opinion to guide us, so our recommendations, given in Figure 8.1, are tentative. Although they are presented in a somewhat linear fashion, we recommend that clinicians consider many of the options simultaneously and use their own judgments regarding appropriate sequencing of queries.

Figure 8.1. A commonsense approach for evaluating "difficult-to-control" hypertension.

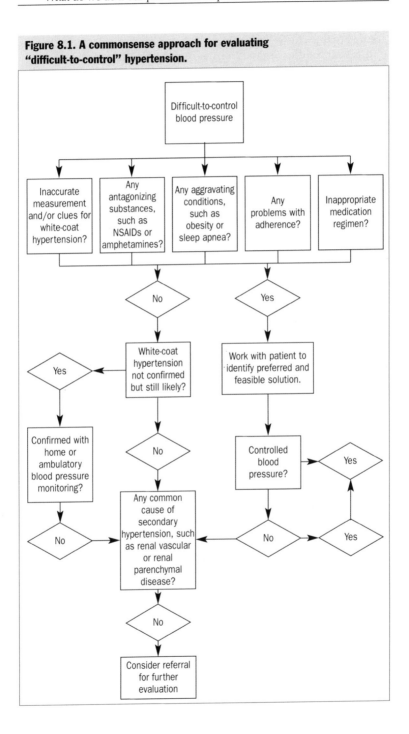

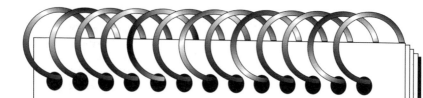

Patient Notes

Mrs Ova Whelms

- Uncontrolled hypertension

Actions

- Blood pressure measurements were repeated with proper technique and confirmed.
- Her drug regimen included 4 drugs at appropriate doses.
- She reported 100% adherence with her medications. She had missed no appointments.

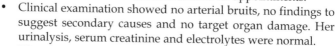

- Clinical examination showed no arterial bruits, no findings to suggest secondary causes and no target organ damage. Her urinalysis, serum creatinine and electrolytes were normal.
- We administered her medications under observation in the office. We gave them in sequence, staggered every 30 minutes to avoid excessive lowering, and measured her blood pressure repeatedly. Her initial reading had been 218/126; two hours later, after one dose of all four drugs, her reading was 174/112.
- We asked her to obtain BP measurements by the office nurse and at a local drugstore and to maintain a log of these readings. She returned with twelve readings documented by others that were consistently elevated to the same range.
- A Doppler ultrasound of her renal arteries showed normal flow bilaterally.
- We changed her to a stronger diuretic, added minoxidil, and her blood pressure began to improve.

Summary bottom lines

- Be alert for patients who fail to achieve treatment targets. (Consensus opinion)

- For most, or even all, such patients, consider the following categories of "difficult-to-control" blood pressure: inaccurate measurement, antagonizing substances such as NSAIDs, coexisting aggravating conditions such as obesity or sleep apnea, suboptimal treatment regimens, and/or nonadherence to treatments. (Consensus opinion)

- For patients whose "difficult-to-control" blood pressure remains unexplained or for patients who have suggestive clues, consider white-coat hypertension (see Chapter 2). Enlist others, such as patients or allied health care professionals, to help monitor blood pressure. If you remain uncertain but suspicious of white-coat hypertension after such measurements, consider ambulatory blood pressure monitoring for confirmation. (Consensus opinion)

- For patients whose resistant hypertension still persists unexplained, or for patients who fit specific patterns of higher risk, consider a selective, sequential evaluation for secondary causes of hypertension. Restrict the initial search to those conditions that are relatively common, such as renovascular causes and renal parenchymal disease. (Consensus opinion)

- Work closely with patients to identify preferred and feasible solutions for correcting any cause of "difficult-to-control" blood pressure that is found. (Consensus opinion)

- For patients with either severe or persistent "difficult-to-control" hypertension, consider referral to centers that specialize in the diagnosis and treatment of resistant hypertension. (Consensus opinion)

We identified information for this chapter by searching MEDLINE 1995 to the present, the Cochrane Controlled Trial Registry and PsycINFO from 1966 to 2000. We hand-searched bibliographies of retrieved articles to find earlier work. We searched for English language, human-related literature relevant to multiple causes of resistant and secondary hypertension. We screened approximately 2500 citations to identify the highest quality, relevant information to include in this chapter.

References

1. Roncaglioni MC, Santoro L, D'Avanzo B, *et al.* Role of family history in patients with myocardial infarction. An Italian case-control study. GISSI-EFRIM Investigators. *Circulation* 1992; **85**:2065-72.

2. Coca A. Actual blood pressure control: are we doing things right? *J Hypertens* 1998; **16** (Suppl):S45-51.

3. Ruilope LM. The hidden truth: what do the clinical trials really tell us about BP control? *J Hum Hypertens* 1995; **9**:S3-7.

4. UK Prospective Diabetes Study Group. Tight blood pressure control and risk of macrovascular and microvascular complications in type 2 diabetes: UKPDS 38 [published erratum appears in *BMJ* 1999; **318**:29]. *BMJ* 1998; **317**:703-13.

5. Yakovlevitch M, Black HR. Resistant hypertension in a tertiary care clinic. *Arch Intern Med* 1991; **151**:1786-92.

6. Williams GH. Hypertensive vascular disease. In: Fauci A, *et al.* editors. *Harrison's principles of internal medicine.* 14th ed. New York: McGraw-Hill, 1998: 1382.

7. Hyman DJ, Pavlik VN. Self-reported hypertension treatment practices among primary care physicians: blood pressure thresholds, drug choices, and the role of guidelines and evidence-based medicine. *Arch Intern Med* 2000; **160**:2281-6.

8. Weir MR, Maibach EW, Bakris GL, *et al.* Implications of a health lifestyle and medication analysis for improving hypertension control. *Arch Intern Med* 2000; **160**:481-90.

9. Gandhi S, Santiesteban H. Resistant hypertension. Suggestions for dealing with the problem. *Postgrad Med* 1996; **100**:97-102,107-8.

10. Setaro JF, Black HR. Refractory hypertension. *N Engl J Med* 1992; **327**:543-7.

11. Oparil S, Calhoun DA. Managing the patient with hard-to-control hypertension. *Am Fam Physician* 1998; **57**:1007-14.

12. Stephenson BJ, Rowe BH, Haynes RB, Macharia WM, Leon G. Is this patient taking the treatment as prescribed? *JAMA* 1993; **269**:2779-81.

13. Baum C, Kennedy DL, Forbes MB. Utilization of nonsteroidal antiinflammatory drugs. *Arthritis Rheum* 1985; **28**:686-92.

14. Houston MC, Weir M, Gray J, *et al.* The effects of nonsteroidal anti-inflammatory drugs on blood pressures of patients with hypertension controlled by verapamil. *Arch Intern Med* 1995; **155**:1049-54.

15. Pope JE, Anderson JJ, Felson DT. A meta-analysis of the effects of nonsteroidal anti-inflammatory drugs on blood pressure. *Arch Intern Med* 1993; **153**:477-84.

16. Johnson AG, Nguyen TV, Day RO. Do nonsteroidal anti-inflammatory drugs affect blood pressure? A meta-analysis. *Ann Intern Med* 1994; **121**:289-300.

17. Brand MB, Mulrow CD, Chiquette E. Weight-reducing diets for control of hypertension in adults. (Cochrane Review) In: *The Cochrane Library, Issue 4*, 1998. Oxford: Update Software.

18. Gifford RW Jr. Evaluation of the hypertensive patient with emphasis on detecting curable causes. *Milbank Mem Fund Q* 1969; **47**:170-86.

19. Tucker RM, Labarthe DR. Frequency of surgical treatment for hypertension in adults at the Mayo Clinic from 1973 through 1975. *Mayo Clin Proc* 1977; **52**:549-55.

20. Davis BA, Crook JE, Vestal RE, Oates JA. Prevalence of renovascular hypertension in patients with grade III or IV hypertensive retinopathy. *N Engl J Med* 1979; **301**:1273-6.

21. Sinclair AM, Isles CG, Brown I, Cameron H, Murray GD, Robertson JW. Secondary hypertension in a blood pressure clinic. *Arch Intern Med* 1987; **147**:1289-93.

22. Lewin A, Blaufox MD, Castle H, Entwisle G, Langford H. Apparent prevalence of curable hypertension in the Hypertension Detection and Follow-up Program. *Arch Intern Med* 1985; **145**:424-7.

23. Kaplan NM, Rose BD. Who should be screened for renovascular or secondary hypertension? [serial online]. *UpToDate.*Version 8.2. Wellesley (MA): UpTo Date, Inc., June 2000.

24. Turnbull JM. Is listening for abdominal bruits useful in the evaluation of hypertension? *JAMA* 1995; **274**:1299-301.

25. Krijnen P, Van Jaarsveld BC, Steyerberg EW, Man In 't Veld AJ, Schalekamp MA, Habbema JD. A clinical prediction rule for renal artery stenosis. *Ann Intern Med* 1998; **129**:705-11.

26. Weber BE, Kapoor WN. Evaluation and outcomes of patients with palpitations. *Am J Med* 1996; **100**:138-48.

27. Grossman EB, Black ER. Secondary hypertension. In: Black ER, Bordley DR, Tape TG, Panzer R, editors. *Diagnostic strategies for common clinical problems.* 2nd ed. Philadelphia (PA): American College of Physicians, 1999.

CHAPTER 9

What if my hypertensive patient becomes pregnant?

Robert L Ferrer
Cynthia D Mulrow

Why is knowledge of hypertension management during pregnancy important?

How do we diagnose hypertension during pregnancy?

What are the maternal and fetal risks for pregnant women with chronic hypertension?

What are the therapeutic options for women with chronic hypertension who are considering pregnancy?

What are the therapeutic options for pregnant women with chronic hypertension?

Does nonpharmacological management of hypertension during pregnancy improve outcomes?

What are the potential benefits of antihypertensive drug therapy for pregnant women with chronic hypertension?

What are the harms of antihypertensive treatment during pregnancy?

How do we weigh the potential benefits and harms of antihypertensive drug treatment during pregnancy?

What are the potential benefits of aspirin for hypertensive pregnant women?

Are there particular monitoring strategies during pregnancy that are warranted or proven beneficial for mothers or fetuses?

Summary bottom lines

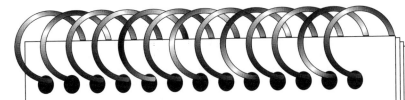

Patient Notes

Mrs Carrie Child, age 36, writer

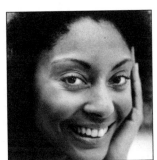

- Controlled hypertension for five years
- 20% overweight
- Takes hydrochlorothiazide and an ACE inhibitor daily

Reason for visit

- She and her husband are considering a second pregnancy.

Clinical questions

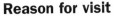

- What are the maternal and fetal risks associated with hypertension during pregnancy?
- Should I modify Mrs Child's current treatment plan for hypertension due to a pending pregnancy?

Why is knowledge of hypertension management during pregnancy important?

Evaluating the obstetrical risks for women with chronic hypertension will become an increasingly common task for clinicians in the coming years because more women are postponing pregnancy and childbirth until the ages when hypertension is more prevalent (Table 9.1). While birth rates at younger ages have been steady or falling, the birth rates for American women over age 30 have increased more than 50% since 1975. For example, 6% of women with first births were older than age 30 in 1975; this statistic had increased to 16% by 1985 and 23% by 1997.[1]

Table 9.1. Prevalence of hypertension among American women 1988 though 1994.[2]

Age	Self-reported hypertension (%)
20 to 24	8.7
25 to 29	12.7
30 to 34	11.0
35 to 39	14.3
40 to 44	17.9

How do we diagnose hypertension during pregnancy?

In most women, the diagnosis of chronic hypertension already will have been made prior to pregnancy, but chronic hypertension also can be diagnosed during pregnancy. As in nonpregnant individuals, neither the distribution of blood pressure among pregnant women nor the relationships between blood pressure levels and maternal and fetal risks provide justification for a rigid separation between normotension and hypertension. Consensus guidelines recommend the following definition for chronic hypertension in pregnancy: blood pressure levels greater than 140/90 mm Hg before 20 weeks' gestation or, belatedly, if hypertension persists more than six weeks after delivery. Hypertension is classified as mild if blood pressure is less than 160/110 mm Hg or as severe if higher.[3]

Hemodynamic changes in pregnancy may affect blood pressure measurement. There are increased distances between Phase IV and V Korotkoff sounds. In up to 7% of normotensive pregnant women, the

Phase V diastolic pressure is 0 mm Hg.[4] In these cases, Phase IV is used to determine diastolic blood pressure. During most pregnancies, there is a physiological fall in diastolic blood pressure that averages 7 to 10 mm Hg and reaches its nadir at about 16 weeks' gestation. This fall in blood pressure is accentuated in hypertensive women.[5]

What are the maternal and fetal risks for pregnant women with chronic hypertension?

We found chronic hypertension is associated with modest increased risk to both the mother and her baby. Potential complications include stillbirth, placental abruption, superimposed preeclampsia, fetal growth restriction, and preterm delivery.

Perinatal mortality

We conducted a systematic review of observational studies comparing mothers with chronic hypertension to normotensive mothers or to general obstetrical populations.[6] The studies consistently showed increased risk of perinatal death with higher compared to lower maternal blood pressures (summary odds ratio 3.4, 95% CI 3.0 to 3.7) (Figure 9.1).[6](Pr: L2, L3) More severe maternal hypertension was associated with greater perinatal mortality than mild to moderate hypertension.[7, 8, 9](Pr: L2b or lower)

Placental abruption

We found observational studies that suggested the risk of placental abruption was increased in women with chronic hypertension (summary odds ratio 2.0; 95% CI 1.1 to 3.7), even after adjusting for sociodemographic factors, smoking status, and parity.[6, 10-12] We found one large retrospective cohort study and one reanalysis of data from a large randomized controlled trial showed that chronic hypertension with superimposed preeclampsia was associated with higher risks of abruption than chronic hypertension alone.[13, 14](Pr: L2b or lower)

Preeclampsia

We found that all but one[15] of six observational studies found positive associations between chronic hypertension and preeclampsia. Actual risk estimates varied, probably because of varying definitions of preeclampsia.[6](Pr: L2b or lower)

Fetal growth

We found 18 observational studies that evaluated risks of prematurity, small-for-gestational-age birthweight, low birthweight, or intrauterine growth restriction associated with chronic hypertension compared to either the general obstetrical population or normotensive pregnant women.[6](Pr: L2b or lower) In all but two studies, chronic hypertension was associated with increased risks of these outcomes. More severe hypertension was associated with more small-for-gestational-age babies than mild to moderate hypertension.

Maternal mortality

We found one large retrospective analysis of a prospectively maintained perinatal database in the United States that examined maternal mortality associated with chronic hypertension.[16](Pr: L2c) In this study, chronic hypertension was defined as blood pressure greater than 140/90 mm Hg occurring earlier than the 20th week of gestation or prepregnancy. The reported maternal mortality among chronic hypertensive pregnant women was 230 out of 100 000 live births. Mortality among normotensive pregnant women was 106 out of 100 000 live births.

Figure 9.1. Perinatal death outcomes from observational studies given as the relative risk (log scale) of women with chronic hypertension compared with either normotensive or general obstetrical populations.[6]

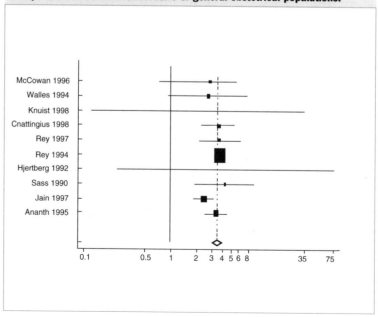

What are the therapeutic options for women with chronic hypertension who are considering pregnancy?

The goals of managing chronic hypertension in women who are seeking to become pregnant are to lower their risk of cardiovascular disease and optimize pregnancy outcomes. We found only scant information regarding these issues. First, we were unable to find any data that related pregnancy outcomes to preconception management of hypertension. Second, we found that the benefits of antihypertensive drug therapy for young women of childbearing age are not precisely known.

We found pooled data regarding cardiovascular morbidity and mortality outcomes from three large trials involving several thousand women aged 30 to 54 are available.[17](Tx: IIa) Women aged 30 to 54 receiving active treatment had a 42% reduction in fatal and nonfatal cerebrovascular events (relative risk 0.58; 95% CI 0.36 to 0.67) and a 27% reduction in combined cardiovascular events (relative risk 0.73; 95% CI 0.54 to 0.97) compared with those assigned to placebo or usual care. There were no statistically significant differences in all cause mortality or fatal cardiovascular or fatal cerebrovascular events. Fewer than 2% of women assigned to the control groups had a fatal or nonfatal cardiovascular event during four to five years of follow-up.

Using above data, the estimated number of nonpregnant, hypertensive women aged 30 to 54 who would need to be treated for five years to prevent a cardiovascular event is approximately 250 (95% CI 158 to 1606). Because this estimate is based on women aged 30 to 54, the number-needed-to-treat would be even higher in most maternity populations, where fewer than one in 1000 births are to women over the age of 45. If we assume an annual risk of a cardiovascular event of less than 0.5% (a safe assumption for most women of childbearing age with mild to moderate chronic hypertension) and that relative risk reductions established in trials are relatively stable, approximately 8000 women of childbearing age would need to be treated annually to prevent one cardiovascular event (95% CI 2500 to 50000). Whether potential benefits of this small magnitude are worth the risks and costs of antihypertensive therapy is a judgment decision best based on individual preferences and values.

What are the therapeutic options for pregnant women with chronic hypertension?

Consensus guidelines recommend drug treatment for severe hypertension in pregnancy (greater than 160/110 mm Hg) to reduce the risk of short-term maternal morbidity. We found that suggestions for managing mild chronic hypertension have been much more controversial, with different national organizations and authorities recommending different treatments and cut-offs and various drugs that are to be favored or shunned.[3, 18-23] Next, we review evidence regarding nonpharmacological treatment, antihypertensive drug therapy, and aspirin prophylaxis.

Does nonpharmacological management of hypertension during pregnancy improve outcomes?

We found consensus guidelines often recommend nonpharmacological therapy, such as activity restriction, bedrest, and calcium supplements, for treating chronic hypertension during pregnancy.[3, 19, 22] We did not identify any controlled studies that evaluated the benefit or harm of nonpharmacological management of chronic hypertension in pregnancy.

What are the potential benefits of antihypertensive drug therapy for pregnant women with chronic hypertension?

We found that treating hypertensive pregnant women with antihypertensive agents reduced intermediate outcomes, such as progression to severe hypertension and the need for adding additional antihypertensives.[6](Tx: L2b) We found that evidence was inconclusive regarding whether drug treatment improved outcomes such as perinatal death, abruption, and fetal growth restriction.

We found 13 small trials involving only 1055 pregnant women that evaluated antihypertensive treatment in pregnant women with mild to moderate chronic hypertension.[6](Tx: LIb, L2b) Six of the trials were placebo-controlled, and seven had a no-treatment group. Eleven different drug regimens were used in the trials. The most commonly studied drug, methyldopa, was given to just over 200 participants.

Data from the trials, presented in Figures 9.2 through 9.4, did not adequately establish or exclude moderate (20 to 50%) effects on most clinical outcomes.[6] One trial found that treating patients with ketanserin plus aspirin lowered the incidence of preeclampsia (4% versus 28%) and placental abruption (9% versus 1%) when compared to aspirin alone.[24](Tx: L2b) One trial reported marked reductions in average birthweights among women given atenolol compared with placebo (2620 versus 3530 grams).[25](Tx: L2b) Small trials that evaluated agents such as methyldopa, hydralazine, labetolol, and thiazide diuretics found no large differences in infant birthweights or risk of small-for-gestational-age infants, or both between treated and untreated mothers (Figure 9.4).

We found a meta-regression of 45 randomized trials that raised further questions about the effect of antihypertensive drug treatment on fetal growth.[26](H: Level not classifiable) These trials enrolled women with pregnancy-induced hypertension as well as women with chronic hypertension. Averaged across trials, a mean fall in mean arterial pressure of 10 mm Hg was associated with a 145-gram reduction in mean birthweight and a higher proportion of small-for-gestational-age infants.[26] Sixteen percent of the variability in birthweight was accounted for by blood pressure. We were uncertain about the clinical significance of the observed small reductions in birthweight, but these data alert us to the possible, but unproven, hypothesis that antihypertensive therapy during pregnancy is more harmful than beneficial.

What are the harms of antihypertensive treatment during pregnancy?

We found little clinical trial evidence regarding harms of specific antihypertensive drug regimens during pregnancy. For example, methyldopa, the most commonly prescribed drug for hypertension in pregnancy, has been used in just over 500 women in clinical trials (including women with pregnancy-induced hypertension). Only two other drugs, labetalol and diuretics, have been used in more than 200 women. Because the clinical trial experience with antihypertensives in pregnancy is so limited, most of the evidence we found on possible adverse effects comes from sources other than clinical trials, such as surveillance studies and case reports. These designs severely limit our ability to calculate the absolute risk of adverse events or to unravel causal relationships.

Figure 9.2. Perinatal death results of trials in pregnant women with mild to moderate chronic hypertension given as risk differences between women assigned to antihypertensive therapy and those assigned to control groups.[6]

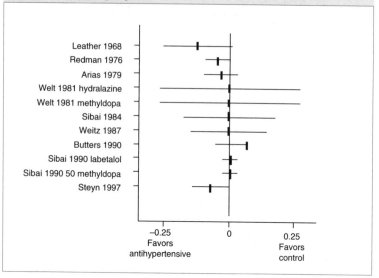

Figure 9.3. Preeclampsia results of trials in pregnant women with mild to moderate chronic hypertension given as risk differences between women assigned to antihypertensive treatment groups and those assigned to control groups.[6]

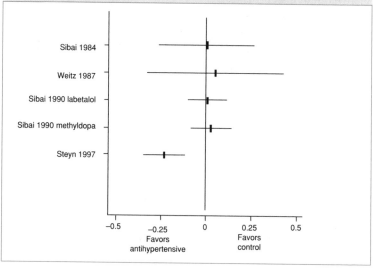

Figure 9.4. Small-for-gestational-age results of trials in pregnant women with mild to moderate chronic hypertension given as risk differences between women assigned to antihypertensive treatment groups and those assigned to control groups.[6]

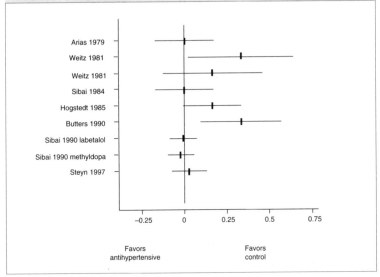

ACE inhibitors probably harmful

We found that the drug class most clearly associated with adverse fetal effects was the ACE inhibitors. They were associated with pulmonary hypoplasia, fetal skull hypoplasia, growth retardation, and fetal renal failure when used in the second and third trimesters,[27-39](H: L4, L5) We were unable to find evidence regarding whether angiotensin II receptor blockers, which act on the same physiological pathway as ACE inhibitors, are also associated with fetal renal failure.

Methyldopa probably safe

We found methyldopa, the antihypertensive almost universally recommended as a first-line agent for treating chronic hypertension in pregnancy, was probably safe for the fetus.[40-42](H: L2b) The most serious risk for the mother was hepatitis. This occurs in the nongravid population at an approximate rate of 1-10000/100000 treated people; it is unknown whether the risk is modified by pregnancy.

Diuretics possibly safe

We found that, despite theoretical concerns about effects of diuretics on plasma volume in pregnancy, findings from a meta-analysis of nine randomized trials and a large cohort study supported their safety.[43, 44](H: L1a, L2b)

Safety unclear for beta-blockers and alpha- and beta-blockers

We found that randomized trials and observational studies reported mixed findings regarding associations between beta-blockers (and alpha- and beta-blockers) and fetal growth restriction.[25, 45-53](H: L2b) Among the beta-blockers studied, atenolol given early in pregnancy was associated with fetal growth restriction in one small trial and two observational studies.[25, 46, 47](H: L2b)

Safety unclear for calcium channel blockers

We found published experience with this class of agents was the most limited of all the classes discussed above.

How do we weigh the potential benefits and harms of antihypertensive drug treatment during pregnancy?

As noted, we found trial data do not adequately prove or disprove the benefits of treating mild to moderate chronic hypertension during pregnancy. Clinicians should consider an individual woman's clinical circumstance and preferences before deciding to initiate or continue antihypertensive therapy during her pregnancy. Next weigh the potential benefits and harms of specific agents to choose the most appropriate therapy. For example, we might choose a particular antihypertensive drug over others if head-to-head comparisons in randomized trials demonstrate its superior efficacy, or, if lacking comparative trials, efficacy is demonstrated in trials for that drug, but not others. Or, in the absence of such trial data, we might choose one drug over others if it has a superior safety record. Conversely, we might avoid particular drugs because of known and possibly severe adverse effects, even if the absolute risk for those effects was unclear.

We found very limited evidence regarding direct comparisons of antihypertensive drugs in trials. We found only two trials that compared different antihypertensive agents in pregnant women with chronic hypertension.[54, 55](Tx: L2b) One involved 300 women and compared methyldopa to labetalol and placebo.[54] No significant differences were reported between the treatment arms in neonatal mortality, birthweight, or Apgar scores. The other trial involved 21 women and compared methyldopa to hydralazine and placebo.[55] No statistically significant differences in pregnancy outcomes were noted. We found neither trial had sufficient power to detect even moderate to large differences in clinically important outcomes.

Until further data become available, we must select a specific antihypertensive drug, if we use one at all, only after weighing estimated or projected relative risks and benefits as derived from various evidence sources. Table 9.2 summarizes the efficacy and harm data presented in previous sections. The antihypertensive agents in the table are those that are specifically recommended or warned against in recent reviews and guidelines.[3, 18-23]

What are the potential benefits of aspirin for hypertensive pregnant women?

We found a review of several randomized trials that evaluated the effect of aspirin prophylaxis among women with a variety of high-risk obstetrical conditions. The trials had variable results, but generally demonstrated no evidence of moderate to large beneficial or harmful effects of aspirin to either the mother or the fetus.[56](Tx: LIa, LIb, L2b) We found 18 randomized trials specifically involving pregnant participants with mild to moderate chronic hypertension and comparing aspirin to either placebo or usual care. These trials consistently showed no moderate to large benefits or harms of aspirin prophylaxis.[6](Tx: LIa, LIb, L2b) We found available trial data were insufficient to rule out some potential benefits of aspirin prophylaxis. For example, the highest quality trial that specifically recruited women with chronic hypertension had 80% power ($p=0.05$) to detect about a 50% relative risk reduction in perinatal mortality, about a 10% to 20% relative risk reduction in preeclampsia, and about a 30% relative risk reduction in intrauterine growth retardation.[57](Tx: L2b) Based on these data, we inform hypertensive women that the benefits and harms of aspirin prophylaxis during their pregnancies are not clearly known but that potential benefits are not likely large.

Table 9.2. Balance sheet of benefits and harms of antihypertensive agents.

Agent or class	Benefits	Harms	Clinical experience in pregnancy
Methyldopa	**Fetal**: Insufficient evidence to rule out large effect on perinatal morbidity or mortality.	**Fetal**: Evidence of no major adverse events.	Large
	Maternal: Insufficient evidence to rule out large effect on maternal morbidity.	**Maternal**: Hepatitis (estimated 1 to 10 per 100 000 in nongravid population).	
Beta-blockers	**Fetal**: Insufficient evidence to ruleout large effect on perinatal morbidity or mortality.	**Fetal**: Limited evidence of possible intrauterine growth retardation if used early in pregnancy.	Large for beta-blockers
Alpha- and beta-blockers	**Maternal**: Insufficient evidence to rule out large effect on maternal morbidity	**Maternal**: Evidence of no major adverse events.	Small for combination alpha- and beta-blockers
Diuretics	**Fetal**: Insufficient evidence to rule out large effect on perinatal morbidity or mortality.	**Fetal**: Evidence of no major adverse events.	Large
	Maternal: Insufficient evidence to rule out large effect on maternal morbidity.	**Maternal**: Evidence of no major adverse events.	
Calcium channel blockers	**Fetal**: Insufficient evidence to rule out large effect on perinatal morbidity or mortality.	**Fetal**: Very limited evidence of no major adverse events.	Small
	Maternal: Insufficient evidence to rule out large effect on maternal morbidity.	**Maternal**: Very limited evidence of no major adverse events.	
Hydralazine	**Fetal**: Insufficient evidence to rule out large effect on perinatal morbidity or mortality.	**Fetal**: Evidence of no major adverse events.	Moderate (for chronic hypertension)
	Maternal: Insufficient evidence to rule out large effect on maternal morbidity.	**Maternal**: Evidence of no major. adverse events.	
ACE inhibitors	**Fetal**: No evidence.	**Fetal**: Risk of fetal renal failure if used in second or third trimester.	Small
Angiotensin II receptor blockers	**Maternal**: No evidence.	**Maternal**: No evidence.	None

Are there particular monitoring strategies during pregnancy that are warranted or proven beneficial for mothers or fetuses?

Women with chronic hypertension in pregnancy are often monitored intensively for maternal and fetal complications, although the benefits, harms, and marginal gains of such monitoring are not clear. Monitoring techniques include serial ultrasonography for fetal growth, Doppler velocimetry of the umbilical or uterine arteries, nonstress tests, biophysical profiles, and biochemical tests, such as plasma urate. We believe that the following are some important issues to consider before using specific monitoring techniques:

- The diagnostic accuracy of the tests for detecting particular maternal and fetal complications

- The efficacy of the monitoring techniques for preventing perinatal morbidity and mortality

- The most effective timing, repeat intervals, and sequencing of tests.

We found no high-level evidence(Level 1, 2, or 3) that examined the accuracy, efficacy, or utility of various different monitoring techniques in pregnant women with chronic hypertension.

Summary bottom lines

- Be aware that more women are postponing pregnancy and childbirth until the ages when hypertension is more prevalent; therefore, evaluating obstetrical risks for women with chronic hypertension will become increasingly important and more frequent.

- Diagnose chronic hypertension in pregnancy when there is known hypertension before pregnancy, blood pressure is over 140/90 before 20 weeks' gestation, or, belatedly, if hypertension persists more than six weeks after delivery. Classify hypertension as mild if blood pressure is less than 160/110 or as severe if higher. (Consensus opinion)

- Inform hypertensive women who are either contemplating pregnancy or pregnant that chronic hypertension is probably associated with increased, but small, absolute risk for both the mother and her baby. Risks may include superimposed preeclampsia, placental abruption, fetal growth restriction, preterm delivery, and stillbirth. (Primarily Level 2 and 3 evidence)

- Inform women of childbearing age that information is scant and

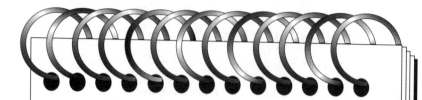

Patient Notes

Mrs Carrie Child

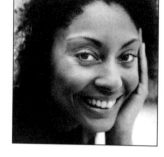

- Controlled hypertension for five years.
- Considering a second pregnancy.

Actions

- Apprise her that hypertension is associated with small absolute increased maternal and fetal risks.
- Apprise her that the benefits and harms of antihypertensive drug therapy during pregnancy are not clear, but pregnancy is probably safe with continued treatement with hydro-chlorothiazide once she becomes pregnant. Also, she should stop taking and avoid ACE inhibitors.
- Refer to a high-risk maternity care provider for management of any future pregnancy.
- Apprise her that she should discuss potential benefits and harms of aspirin prophylaxis with the high-risk maternity care provider but that benefits are unlikely large.

imprecise regarding whether and how to lower their own risk of cardiovascular disease attributable to hypertension. Use the risk equations discussed in Chapter 3 to advise them of their individual risks of cardiovascular disease over the next one to five years. For most women contemplating pregnancy, these risks will be very low. Use the following relative risk, derived from trial data in hypertensive women aged 30 to 54, to estimate the reduction in cardiovascular events that might be expected with short and intermediate-term antihypertensive therapy: relative risk 0.73, 95% CI 0.54 to 0.97. In general, several thousand women of childbearing age would need to be treated for one year in order to prevent one cardiovascular event. (Extrapolation of Level 1 and 2 evidence)

- Inform hypertensive pregnant women with mild to moderate hypertension that there is little known benefit of antihypertensive treatment during pregnancy. (Lack of Level 1 evidence) Potential benefits are prevention of severe hypertension during pregnancy. (Level 2 evidence) Whether antihypertensive treatment could decrease uncommon outcomes such as perinatal death, abruption, or clinically significant fetal growth restriction is unknown. (Mixed Level 2 evidence)

- Inform women who are either contemplating pregnancy or pregnant that ACE inhibitors should be avoided because they may be associated with fetal abnormalities such as renal failure. (Level 4 evidence) Inform women that diuretics and methyldopa appear safe because they have not been associated with major fetal abnormalities. (Level 1 and 2 evidence) Inform women that beta-blockers and combination alpha- and beta-blockers may increase risk of fetal growth restriction, although evidence is scant and conflicting. (Mixed Level 2 evidence) Inform women that knowledge of risks associated with other agents, such as calcium channel blockers, is very limited.

- Consider using simple balance sheets, such as the one given in Table 9.2, to help women understand the largely unknown, but potential, benefits and harms of antihypertensive therapies for themselves and their babies. (Opinion)

- Inform women that the benefits and harms of nonpharmacological management of chronic hypertension in pregnancy are unknown. (Lack of Level 1 and 2 evidence)

- Inform hypertensive pregnant women that little is known about the benefits and harms of various monitoring strategies, such as serial ultrasonography for fetal growth, Doppler velocimetry of the umbilical or uterine arteries, nonstress tests, biophysical profiles, and biochemical tests such as plasma urate. (Lack of Level 1 and 2 evidence)

* Inform hypertensive women that the benefits and harms of aspirin prophylaxis during their pregnancies are not clearly known but that potential benefits are not likely large. (Level 1 and 2 evidence)

We identified information for this chapter by searching 16 electronic databases from 1966 to 1999 and MEDLINE from 1999 to 2000. The 16 electronic databases included, but were not limited to, MEDLINE, EMBASE, the Cochrane Controlled Trial Register and Pregnancy and Childbirth Database, CINAHL, REPROTOX, TERIS, and the Motherrisk Program. We used four general search strategies to identify English and non-English language, human-related literature relevant to antihypertensive treatment efficacy during pregnancy, harms of specific antihypertensive agents, fetal and maternal risks associated with maternal elevations in blood pressure, and specific monitoring techniques. We screened more than 6000 titles and/or abstracts to help identify the highest quality relevant information to include in the chapter. Of note, work for this chapter was funded by a grant from the Agency for Healthcare Research and Quality to the San Antonio Evidence-Based Practice Center.

References

1. Ventura SJ, Mosher WD, Curtin SC, Abma JC, Henshaw S. Trends in pregnancies and pregnancy rates by outcome: estimates for the United States, 1976-96. *Vital Health Stat* 2000; **21**:1-47.

2. National Center for Health Statistics (US). *National Health and Examination Survey III, 1988-94.* Version 1.22a, rev. Oct 1997. Hyattsville (MD): US Dept of Health and Human Services, Centers for Disease Control and Prevention, National Center for Health Statistics, 1997.

3. National High Blood Pressure Education Program Working Group. National High Blood Pressure Education Program Working Group Report on High Blood Pressure in Pregnancy. *Am J Obstet Gynecol* 1990; **163**:1691-712.

4. Wichman K, Ryden G, Wichman M. The influence of different positions and Korotkoff sounds on the blood pressure measurements in pregnancy. *Acta Obstet Gynecol Scand* 1984; **118**(Suppl):25-8.

5. Chesley LC, Annitto JE. Pregnancy in the patient with hypertensive disease. *Am J Obstet Gynecol* 1947; **53**:372-81.

6. Ferrer RL, Sibai BM, Mulrow CD, Chiquette E, Stevens KR, Cornell J. Management of mild chronic hypertension during pregnancy: a review. *Obstet Gynecol* 2000; **96**: 849-60.

7. Sass N, Moron AF, El-Kadre D, Camano L, De Almeida PA. [Study of pregnancy with chronic hypertension]. [Portuguese]. *Rev Paul Med* 1990; **108**:261-6.

8. Curet LB, Olson RW. Evaluation of a program of bed rest in the treatment of chronic hypertension in pregnancy. *Obstet Gynecol* 1979; **53**:336-40.

9. Dunlop JC. Chronic hypertension and perinatal mortality. *Proc R Soc Med* 1966; **59**:838-41.

10. Williams MA, Mittendorf R, Monson RR. Chronic hypertension, cigarette smoking, and abruptio placentae. *Epidemiology* 1991; **2**:450-3.

11. Ananth CV, Bowes WA Jr, Savitz DA, Luther ER. Relationship between pregnancy-induced hypertension and placenta previa: a population-based study. *Am J Obstet Gynecol* 1997; **177**:997-1002.

12. Kramer MS, Usher RH, Pollack R, Boyd M, Usher S. Etiologic determinants of abruptio placentae. *Obstet Gynecol* 1997; **89**:221-6.

13. Sibai BM, Lindheimer M, Hauth J, *et al.* Risk factors for preeclampsia, abruptio placentae, and adverse neonatal outcomes among women with chronic hypertension. National Institute of Child Health and Human Development Network of Maternal-Fetal Medicine Units. *N Engl J Med* 1998; **339**:667-71.

14. Ananth CV, Savitz DA, Bowes WA Jr, Luther ER. Influence of hypertensive disorders and cigarette smoking on placental abruption and uterine bleeding during pregnancy. *Br J Obstet Gynaecol* 1997; **104**:572-8.

15. Sibai BM, Abdella TN, Anderson GD. Pregnancy outcome in 211 patients with mild chronic hypertension. *Obstet Gynecol* 1983; **61**:571-6.

16. Jain L. Effect of pregnancy-induced and chronic hypertension on pregnancy outcome. *J Perinatol* 1997; **17**:425-7.

17. Quan A, Kerlikowske K, Gueyffier F, Boissel JP. Efficacy of treating hypertension in women. *J Gen Intern Med* 1999; **14**:718-29.

18. Witlin AG, Sibai BM. Hypertension. *Clin Obstet Gynecol* 1998; **41**:533-44.

19. Perloff D. Hypertension and pregnancy-related hypertension. *Cardiol Clin* 1998; **16**:79-101.

20. Rey E, LeLorier J, Burgess E, Lange IR, Leduc L. Report of the Canadian Hypertension Society Consensus Conference: 3. Pharmacologic treatment of hypertensive disorders in pregnancy. *CMAJ* 1997; **157**:1245-54.

21. Paller MS. Hypertension in pregnancy. *J Am Soc Nephrol* 1998; **9**:314-21.

22. Neerhof MG. Pregnancy in the chronically hypertensive patient. *Clin Perinatol* 1997; **24**:391-406.

23. Khedun SM, Moodley J, Naicker T, Maharaj B. Drug management of hypertensive disorders of pregnancy. *Pharmacol Ther* 1997; **74**:221-58.

24. Steyn DW, Odendaal HJ. Randomised controlled trial of ketanserin and aspirin in prevention of pre-eclampsia. *Lancet* 1997; **350**:1267-71.

25. Butters L, Kennedy S, Rubin PC. Atenolol in essential hypertension during pregnancy. *BMJ* 1990; **301**:587-9.

26. Von Dadelszen P, Ornstein MP, Bull SB, Logan AG, Koren G, Magee LA. Fall in mean arterial pressure and fetal growth restriction in pregnancy hypertension: a meta-analysis. *Lancet* 2000; **355**:87-92.

27. Duminy PC, Burger PD. Fetal abnormality associated with the use of captopril during pregnancy. *S Afr Med J* 1981; **60**:805.

28. Barr M Jr, Cohen MM Jr. ACE inhibitor fetopathy and hypocalvaria: the kidney-skull connection. *Teratology* 1991; **44**:485-95.

29. Hanssens M, Keirse MJ, Vankelecom F, Van Assche FA. Fetal and neonatal effects of treatment with angiotensin-converting enzyme inhibitors in pregnancy. *Obstet Gynecol* 1991; **78**:128-35.

30. Pryde PG, Sedman AB, Nugent CE, Barr M Jr. Angiotensin-converting enzyme inhibitor fetopathy. *J Am Soc Nephrol* 1993; **3**:1575-82.

31. Piper JM, Ray WA, Rosa FW. Pregnancy outcome following exposure to angiotensin-converting enzyme inhibitors. *Obstet Gynecol* 1992; **80**:429-32.

32. Cunniff C, Jones KL, Phillipson J, Benirschke K, Short S, Wujek J. Oligohydramnios sequence and renal tubular malformation associated with maternal enalapril use. *Am J Obstet Gynecol* 1990; **162**:187-9.

33. Bhatt-Mehta V, Deluga KS. Fetal exposure to lisinopril: neonatal manifestations and management. *Pharmacotherapy* 1993; **13**:515-18.

34. Lavoratti G, Seracini D, Fiorini P, *et al.* Neonatal anuria by ACE inhibitors during pregnancy. *Nephron* 1997; **76**:235-6.

35. Thorpe-Beeston JG, Armar NA, Dancy M, Cochrane GW, Ryan G, Rodeck CH. Pregnancy and ACE inhibitors. *Br J Obstet Gynaecol* 1993; **100**:692-3.

36. Chisholm CA, Chescheir NC, Kennedy M. Reversible oligohydramnios in a pregnancy with angiotensin-converting enzyme inhibitor exposure. *Am J Perinatol* 1997; **14**:511-13.

37. Sadeck LS, Fernandes M, Silva SM, *et al.* [Captopril use in pregnancy and its effects on the fetus and the newborn: case report]. [Portuguese]. *Rev Hosp Clin Fac Med Sao Paulo* 1997; **52**:328-32.

38. Centers for Disease Control and Prevention. From the Centers for Disease Control and Prevention. Postmarketing surveillance for angiotensin-converting enzyme inhibitor use during the first trimester of pregnancy – United States, Canada, and Israel, 1987-1995. *JAMA* 1997; **277**:1193-4.

39. Postmarketing surveillance for angiotensin-converting enzyme inhibitor use during the first trimester of pregnancy – United States, Canada, and Israel, 1987-1995. *MMWR* 1997; **46**:240-2.

40. Briggs GG, Freeman RK, Yaffee SJ. *Drugs in pregnancy and lactation: a reference guide to fetal and neonatal risk.* 5th ed. Baltimore (MD): Williams & Wilkins, 1998.

41. Meyler L. *Meyler's side effects of drugs.* 1996 (annual) ed. New York: Excerpta Medica Foundation, 1996.

42. Davies DM. *Textbook of adverse drug reactions.* 4th ed. Oxford; New York: Oxford University Press, 1991.

43. Cuadros A, Tatum HJ. The prophylactic and therapeutic use of bendroflumethizide in pregnancy. *Am J Obstet Gynecol* 1964; **89**:891-7.

44. Christianson R, Page EW. Diuretic drugs and pregnancy. *Obstet Gynecol* 1976; **48**:647-52.

45. Dubois D, Petitcolas J, Temperville B, Klepper A, Catherine P. Beta blocker therapy in 125 cases of hypertension during pregnancy. *Clin Exp Hypertens* [B] 1983; **2**:41-59.

46. Lip GY, Beevers M, Churchill D, Shaffer LM, Beevers DG. Effect of atenolol on birth weight. *Am J Cardiol* 1997; **79**:1436-8.

47. Butters L. Essential hypertension in pregnancy. *Nurs Times* 1990; **86**:53.

48. Montan S, Ingemarsson I, Marsal K, Sjoberg NO. Randomised controlled trial of atenolol and pindolol in human pregnancy: effects on fetal haemodynamics. *BMJ* 1992; **304**:946-9.

49. Tuimala R, Hartikainen-Sorri AL. Randomized comparison of atenolol and pindolol for treatment of hypertension in pregnancy. *Curr Ther Res Clin Exp* 1988; **44**:579-84.

50. Rubin PC, Butters L, Clark D, *et al.* Obstetric aspects of the use in pregnancy-associated hypertension of the beta-adrenoceptor antagonist atenolol. *Am J Obstet Gynecol* 1984; **150**:389-92.

51. Rubin PC, Butters L, Clark DM, *et al.* Placebo-controlled trial of atenolol in treatment of pregnancy-associated hypertension. *Lancet* 1983; i:431-4.

52. Marlettini MG, Crippa S, Morselli-Labate AM, Contarini A, Orlandi C. Randomized comparison of calcium antagonists and beta-blockers in the treatment of pregnancy-induced hypertension. *Curr Ther Res Clin Exp* 1990; **48**:684-94.

53. Fabregues G, Alvarez L, Varas Juri P, *et al.* Effectiveness of atenolol in the treatment of hypertension during pregnancy. *Hypertension* 1992; **19**:II129-31.

54. Sibai BM, Mabie WC, Shamsa F, Villar MA, Anderson GD. A comparison of no medication versus methyldopa or labetalol in chronic hypertension during pregnancy. *Am J Obstet Gynecol* 1990; **162**:960-6.

55. Welt SI, Dorminy JH 3d, Jelovsek FR, Crenshaw MC, Gall SA. The effects of prophylactic management and therapeutics on hypertensive disease in pregnancy: preliminary studies. *Obstet Gynecol* 1981; **57**:557-65.

56. Gallery EDM, Ross MR, Hawkins M, Leslie G, Gyory AZ. Low-dose aspirin in high-risk pregnancy? *Hypertens Preg* 1997; **16**:229-38.

57. Caritis S, Sibai B, Hauth J, *et al*. Low-dose aspirin to prevent preeclampsia in women at high risk. National Institute of Child Health and Human Development Network of Maternal-Fetal Medicine Units. *N Engl J Med* 1998; **338**:701-5.

Index